Coagulation Disorders - Innovative Developments in Diagnostic and Therapeutic Approaches

Edited by Cees Th. Smit Sibinga

Published in London, United Kingdom

Coagulation Disorders - Innovative Developments in Diagnostic and Therapeutic Approaches
http://dx.doi.org/10.5772/intechopen.1003491
Edited by Cees Th. Smit Sibinga

Contributors
Alexy Maza Villadiego, Antonio Ciampa, Cem Selim, Elena Tuna Aguilar, Mariachiara Gagliardi, Mariem Pulido Flores, Małgorzata Wiszniewska, Oscar Jaime Moreno García, Samuel Sarmiento Doncel, Ángel Gabriel Vargas Ruiz

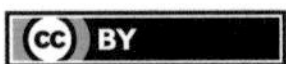

First published in London, United Kingdom, 2025 by IntechOpen
IntechOpen is the global imprint of INTECHOPEN LIMITED, registered in England and Wales, registration number: 11086078, 167-169 Great Portland Street, London, W1W 5PF, United Kingdom

For EU product safety concerns: IN TECH d.o.o., Prolaz Marije Krucifikse Kozulić 3, 51000 Rijeka, Croatia, info@intechopen.com or visit our website at intechopen.com.

British Library Cataloguing-in-Publication Data
A catalogue record for this book is available from the British Library

Coagulation Disorders - Innovative Developments in Diagnostic and Therapeutic Approaches
Edited by Cees Th. Smit Sibinga
p. cm.
Print ISBN 978-0-85466-953-0
Online ISBN 978-0-85466-952-3
eBook (PDF) ISBN 978-0-85466-954-7

If disposing of this product, please recycle the paper responsibly.

Meet the editor

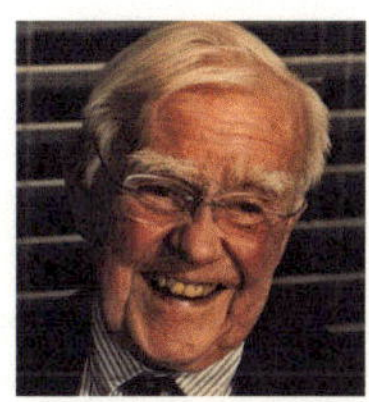

Cees Th. Smit Sibinga is a Clinical Hematologist and Transfusion Medicine Specialist at UMCG, Groningen, and was the Director of the Regional Blood Bank North Nederland (1976–2004). He served as Professor of International Development of Transfusion Medicine at the University of Groningen. Through IQM Consulting, he has been involved in developing Transfusion Medicine and quality systems for economically restricted countries, working with WHO, WFH, and ICBS. He is the founder of the Academic Institute for International Development of Transfusion Medicine (IDTM) at the University of Groningen, focusing on countries with restricted economies. He also established Sanquin (2000), AABB Consulting Services (2001), and the Consulting Service for International Development of Quality Management in Transfusion Medicine (IQM Consulting) (2001). He has organized 28 international scientific symposia on Transfusion Medicine in Groningen, published over 400 peer-reviewed scientific articles and book chapters, and contributed countless peer-reviewed scientific abstracts. Additionally, he has edited over 40 books.

Contents

Preface

Since the innovative mid-19th-century approach of Rudolf Ludwig Carl Virchow and his colleagues at the Charité University Hospital in Berlin on hemostasis and blood coagulation—summarized in the famous Virchow's Triad of thrombosis and blood coagulation (vessel wall, blood flow, and blood composition)—a continuous avalanche of groundbreaking research has emerged worldwide. Robert Gwyn MacFarlane, Armand James Quick, and many other renowned scientists initiated this wave of discoveries.

Blood clotting, or blood coagulation, is an important physiologic and defensive process that prevents excessive bleeding when a blood vessel is injured or when an inherited deficiency of one or more coagulation factors is present like in hemophilia. Platelets or thrombocytes (a type of blood cell) and proteins (clotting factors) in the plasma (the liquid part of the blood) work together to stop the bleeding by forming a fibrin clot over the injury. Platelets or thrombocytes are small, colorless cell fragments without a nucleus of megakaryocytes (in the bone marrow) in the blood that form clots or aggregates and stop or prevent bleeding. Platelets are made in our bone marrow, the sponge-like tissue inside our bones. Bone marrow contains stem cells that develop into red blood cells, white blood cells, and megakaryocytes that produce platelets through karyorrhexis.

Today, the question arises: what is new, and what is still unknown? What clinical phenomena and diseases need a precise diagnosis or innovative diagnostic approach, and what is the underlying pathology or causative metabolic, genetic or biochemical aberration? How can we pinpoint and treat these diseases, pathological phenomena, and aberrations?

Apart from advancements in gene therapy and genetic manipulation, could nanotechnology and well-controlled artificial intelligence enable earlier and more accurate diagnosis, as well as more targeted, effective, and sustained treatments while minimizing unnecessary side effects? Various multidisciplinary research groups and academic institutes are exploring innovative approaches through new inventions and discoveries. They collaborate closely with leading university healthcare institutes, emphasizing the ethical and legal aspects of these advancements. Unfortunately, some developed countries have implemented policies based on decrees that significantly slow scientific progress in these innovative fields, hindering new developments and delaying cutting-edge research intended for the benefit of humanity.

This book highlights several clinical roadblocks through intelligent observations and out-of-the-box thinking, bringing to light innovative advancements in diagnostic and therapeutic approaches within the field of clinical blood coagulation and its overshoot.

Cees Th. Smit Sibinga
IQM Consulting and University of Groningen,
Groningen, The Netherlands

Chapter 1

The Importance of Searching for Acquired von Willebrand Syndrome in Chronic Myeloproliferative Neoplasms

Mariem Pulido Flores, Ángel Gabriel Vargas Ruiz, Oscar Jaime Moreno García and Elena Tuna Aguilar

Abstract

Acquired von Willebrand syndrome is an entity unknown and misdiagnosed in most cases. It is a bleeding disorder presented with mild to moderate hemorrhagic symptoms secondary to lymphoproliferative disorders (and known as the most frequent cause of acquired von Willebrand syndrome), cardiovascular disease, myeloproliferative neoplasms (essential thrombocythemia, polycythemia vera, and chronic myeloid leukemia), autoimmune disease or solid neoplasms. The most known mechanisms of a von Willebrand antigen diminished consist of an increased degradation or clearance of circulating VWF. This occurs due to an increased plasma clearance of von Willebrand factor (VWF) caused by antibodies, cell adsorption, shear stress, or increased proteolysis induced by ADAMTS 13. Diagnosis is made by clinical assessment supplemented by laboratory tests of complete blood count (CBC), PT, aPTT with a VWF antigen, VWF:RCo, high molecular weight (HMW) multimer), and FVIII activity with findings in most cases the ratio of VWF:RCo to VWF:Ag usually diminished (<0.7) with a loss of HMW multimers. Management includes the selection of the best treatment for acute bleeding and treating the underlying condition Acquired von Willebrand syndrome is a pathology that should be investigated in chronic myeloproliferative neoplasms when platelet counts approach one million and the increase in hematocrit is significant, as it predisposes to bleeding.

Keywords: myeloproliferative neoplasms, von Willebrand syndrome, endothelial injury, thrombocytosis, ristocetin cofactor activity (VWF:RCo), ADAMTS13

1. Introduction

Acquired von Willebrand syndrome (AVWS) is a rare but probably underestimated bleeding disorder characterized by laboratory findings and clinical presentations like those of inherited von Willebrand disease (VWD), which is classified in quantitative (types 1 and 3) or qualitative (type 2) defects in von Willebrand factor

(VWF). Compared with von Willebrand disease, AVWS usually occurs in adults with no personal family or history of a bleeding diathesis [1].

The first case of acquired von Willebrand syndrome was described in 1962 in a boy with systemic lupus erythematosus [2]. Through time, AVWS has been associated with other diseases, including lymphoproliferative disorders, autoimmune disorders, structural heart diseases including aortic stenosis, congenital heart defects, and the use of left ventricular assist devices or extracorporeal membrane oxygenation (ECMO); and myeloproliferative neoplasms (MPN), mainly in essential thrombocythemia (ET) and polycythemia vera (PV) [1, 3, 4].

Lymphoproliferative disorders are the most common underlying disease associated with AVWS in 70%; the majority of cases described are non-Hodgkin lymphoma and plasma cell dyscrasias, followed by heart defects and myeloproliferative neoplasms with 10–70% and 10–20%, respectively. Other less common diseases associated with AVWS include Wilms tumor, hypothyroidism, and autoimmune disorders [5, 6].

2. Understanding acquired von Willebrand syndrome in myeloproliferative neoplasms

Von Willebrand factor (VWF) is a multimeric plasma glycoprotein synthesized by endothelial cells and megakaryocytes, which promotes platelet adhesion and aggregation at the site of vascular injury where it forms an adhesive bridge between platelets and the endothelial surface, especially in areas of high shear stress, significantly contributing for primary hemostasis (**Figure 1**) [1].

AVWS in patients with MPN results from the loss of high molecular weight VWF multimers. Mechanisms that have been found to explain this include autoantibodies production against von Willebrand factor and a high shear stress due to a high hematocrit and high platelet counts found in MPN [3].

AVWS in myeloproliferative neoplasms presents with platelet counts above $500x10^9/L$, however, diagnosis is made in most cases when the platelet count is more than $1000x10^9/L$ [6].

Certain driver gene mutations in MPN like Janus kinase 2 (*JAK2 V617F*), calreticulin (*CALR*), or thrombopoietin receptor (*MPL*) are found in most of the cases, with *JAK2 V617F* the most related driver gene mutation in myeloproliferative neoplasms, including polycythemia vera, essential thrombocythemia, and primary myelofibrosis. *JAK2 V617F* mutation has the most high-risk profile for thrombosis in MPN. One hundred sixteen patients review of factors related to the development of AVWS in patients with essential thrombocythemia and polycythemia vera, found *JAK2 V617F* as an independent risk factor for the development of AVWS. In addition, VWF:RCo levels and the VWF:RCo/VWF:Ag ratio were significantly lower among *JAK2 V617F* positive ET patients. ET patients harboring the *JAK2 V617F* mutation were significantly more likely to develop AVWS than CALR-positive patients, despite significantly lower platelet counts [6].

Essential thrombocythemia is considered the underlying disease most related to AVWS, followed by polycythemia vera and primary myelofibrosis in third place. Also, a high hematocrit in MPN, specifically in PV plays an essential role in the development of AVWS. High hematocrit influences blood rheology, thereby increasing shear stress values [3]. The increased shear stress may induce a conformational change in the VWF molecule, enabling its interaction with its platelet receptor (i.e., Gplb) and its proteolysis by ADAMTS13 (a disintegrin-like and metalloprotease with thrombospondin type 1 motif no. 13) [7].

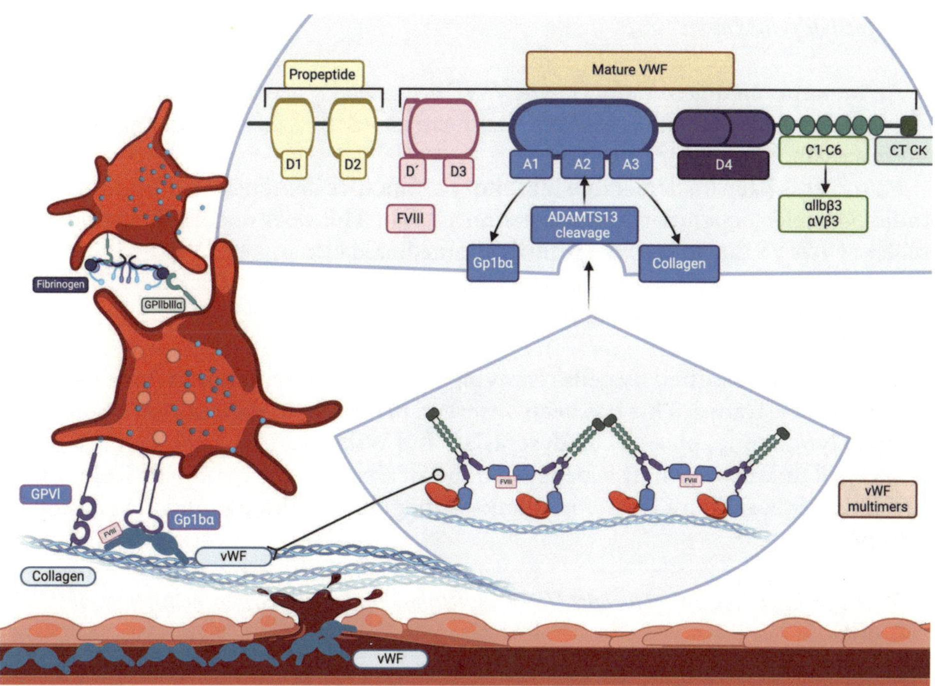

Figure 1.
Functions of von Willebrand factor. Dimeric subunits of von Willebrand factor undergo multimerization, multimers will be stored in Weibel-Palade bodies in endothelial cells and α -granules of the platelets. Multimers of VWF and collagen fibers are released when endothelial damage occurs. High molecular weight VWF multimers provide multiple binding sites that can interact with platelets and the subendothelium, promoting platelet adhesion for primary hemostasis. Several proteases can cleave VWF, including ADAMTS13 in domain A2 of VWF which plays an essential role in promoting VWF clearance. Although, VWF acts as a protective carrier protein for FVIII, contributing to clot formation by maintaining regular FVIII levels.

2.1 Clinical features

The main clinical features include mild to moderately severe mucocutaneous bleeding (ecchymosis, epistaxis, menorrhagia, gastrointestinal tract bleeding) and bleeding diathesis that usually occurs late in life in persons with non-past and family history of bleeding [8].

Gastrointestinal bleeding is common in patients with AVWS, and it is associated with the detection of angiodysplasia, explained by the theory of increased angiogenesis due to an increased clearance of VWF. Gastrointestinal bleeding can be present as Heyde syndrome, which is characterized by AVWS with cardiovascular disorders such as aortic stenosis or severe mitral regurgitation [9, 10].

2.2 Pathophysiology

High molecular weight multimers of the von Willebrand factor are the most active functional form of the molecule, and they have different binding sites for platelets and subendothelial molecules. Consequently, VWF depletion, particularly of high molecular weight multimers, can cause mucocutaneous hemorrhage and arteriovenous malformations [3].

Unlike acquired hemophilia, the complex pathophysiology of AVWS involves different mechanisms described below:

2.2.1 Antibody-mediated

An immune-mediated reduction of VWF is caused by the formation of specific or non-specific auto-antibodies to VWF that form circulating immune complexes with and inactivate VWF [11].

Many cases have no detectable inhibitory antibodies demonstrated by admixture studies (platelet-dependent VWF function assays). This does not eliminate the possibility of AWVS due to increased antibody-mediated clearance of VWF [5].

2.2.2 Adsorption of VWF onto malignant cell clones

VWF can be absorbed by cells removing it from the circulation, which will lead to increased clearance. This has been observed primarily in patients with non-Hodgkin lymphoma, plasma cell dyscrasias, and Wilms tumor. The exact mechanism is still unknown, but it is believed to be an aberrant expression of Gplb. This mechanism is seen more frequently in non-Hodgkin lymphomas and plasma cell dyscrasias [12, 13].

2.2.3 Loss of high molecular weight VWF multimers under conditions of high shear stress

The multimeric structure of VWF makes the protein sensitive to changes in fluid flow and shear stress, and in normal circulation, VWF tumbles and undergoes oscillatory force cycles every few milliseconds in areas of high shear stress, VWF multimers that become unfolded and more elongated are the more susceptible for cleavage by ADAMTS13. This mechanism can be seen in increased shear stress pathologies such as ventricular septal defect, valvulopathies, ECMO, and left ventricular assist devices [14].

2.2.4 Increased proteolytic degradation of VWF by circulating proteases

An increased VWF degradation from leukocyte-derived serine proteases can also hypothesized because cathepsin G, elastase, and proteinase 3 could cleave VWF similarly to ADAMTS13. Increased proteolysis has been seen in multiple myeloma and essential thrombocythemia [15].

The increased clearance of VWF follows an FVIII deficiency, whereas VWF acts as a carrier protein for factor VIIl. Factor VIII deficiency is usually seen in moderate to severe AVWS. Decreased FVIII may contribute to muscle or joint bleeding.

3. When to suspect AVWS in myeloproliferative neoplasms

The first step to be considered is the absence of a family history of bleeding. The laboratory tests are the same as those used to diagnose inherited von Willebrand disease [16].

The best screening remains the patient's medical history, including personal and family history of abnormal bleeding and hemostatic challenges [6].

VWF levels should be considered if the AVWS suspicion is high, and in individuals with MPN where the administration of aspirin is part of the standard treatment.

3.1 Diagnosis of AVWS

A platelet-dependent von Willebrand factor activity test and its relationship to the antigen are used for diagnosis. It can be VWF: Ristocetin Cofactor/VWF Antigen ratio (VWF: RCo/VWF Ag) or VWF antigen (VWF: Gplb or VWF: RCo/VWF: Ag) but the relationship can also be used or VWF: Collagen Binding/VWF Antigen ratio (VWF CB/VWF Ag) [16].

A high VWF: propeptide to VWF:Ag ratio indicates increased clearance of VWF, which can be helpful in both the diagnosis and in confirming remission after treatment [6]. Definitive reference ranges that specifically define AVWS have not been established, considering the cut-off values for VWD as a reasonable approach to AVWS diagnosis, finding in most cases platelet-dependent VWF activity to VWF antigen (VWF:Gplb or VWF:RCo/VWF:Ag) diminished (ratio < 0.7), same values for diagnosis found in type 2 VWD [8].

Distinguishing AVWS from VWD should be done for treatment decisions and for searching for an underlying disease of AVWS and early treatment. The main clinical features and personal history for guiding AVWS diagnosis are the following:

- Late onset of bleeding, no uneventful surgery, or no previous high-risk situations.
- Negative bleeding family history or congenital bleeding disease (VWD)
- An AVWS-associated disorder (heart defects, lymphoproliferative disorder, myeloproliferative neoplasms, autoimmune disorders, hypothyroidism, solid tumor).
- Presence of inhibitor or VWF binding antibodies.
- Remission after treatment of underlying disorder; response to IVIG in IgG Monoclonal Gammopathy of Undetermined Significance (MGUS)-associated with AVWS.
- Short-lived response to VWF containing concentrates or desmopressin [16].

In AVWS, there may be a deficiency of high and intermediate molecular weight multimers of the von Willebrand factor, similar to VWD type 2A.

Current guidelines for the treatment of ET recommend the routine assessment of ristocetin cofactor activity (VWF:RCo) in ET patients with platelet counts above $1000 \times 10^9/L$ and to withhold aspirin for cardiovascular prevention if VWF:RCo is <30% [17, 18].

4. Treatment in AVWS

Evaluation and management of von Willebrand syndrome may be complex, especially in those for whom the underlying disorder requires antithrombotic therapy, such as anticoagulation for a prosthetic heart valve or aspirin use for essential thrombocythemia.

The goals of treatment in AVWS are to control recurrent bleeding episodes, to prevent bleeding when an invasive procedure is necessary, and, when possible, to control the underlying disease [16].

Various therapeutic approaches have been used to treat patients with AVWS, including desmopressin (dDAVP), VWF concentrates, high-dose intravenous immunoglobulin (IVIG), plasmapheresis, corticosteroids, and immune suppressive drugs [16].

4.1 Desmopressin

The dDAVP promotes the release of VWF from Weibel-Palade bodies into circulation. This VWF could reduce bleeding due to its hemostatic effect compared to the circulating von Willebrand factor in AVWS, which binds to autoantibodies in an inactive form. Desmopressin has a short-lasting action, necessitating adjacent treatment with a long-acting drug that reduces circulating vWF antibodies [9].

In the ISTH registry, an overall success rate of 32% was observed with the use of desmopressin, but that rates varied according to the underlying disorder, being low in cardiovascular disease (10%), myeloproliferative neoplasm (21%) and autoimmune disorders (33%) but being higher in lymphoproliferative disorders (44%) and neoplastic disorders (75%) [19]. The most common adverse effect of the use of desmopressin, especially when heart defects remain the underlying disease, is hyponatremia due to high fluid overload [9].

4.2 Intravenous immunoglobulin

The therapeutic doses of IVIG for AVWS are 1 g/kg per day for 2 days or 0.4 g/kg per day for 5 days, as proposed for immune primary thrombocytopenia.

As IVIG usually requires 24–48 h to normalize plasma VWF/FVIII activity, they induced a prompt and sustained increase of VWF activity and shortening of bleeding time in patients with AVWS associated with IgG–MGUS, although patients with paraproteins of the IgM class do not respond to IVIG, the use of plasmapheresis has been effective [20].

Repeated doses of IVIG given every 21 days (long-term therapy) can produce consistent responses in VWF measurements, but high doses seem critical for IVIG effects [6].

4.3 Other non-specific therapies

Recombinant factor VIIa (rVIIa) is used when bleeding associated with AVWS is unresponsive to standard therapy [21].

VWF concentrates are used for clinically significant bleeding. VWF concentrates are IV administered after a poor response to a therapeutic trial with dDAVP, or sometimes initially, depending on availability and circumstances.

Recombinant VWF (rVWF) is useful because of its long half-life. It is important to obtain levels of VWF and FVIII activity immediately before and following infusion to determine the half-life of the infused products. Post-infusion levels can be measured at 4, 8, and 12 hours after the first infusion to obtain half-life information of rVWF.

4.4 Treatment in myeloproliferative neoplasms

Treatment of MPN should remove the AVWS, and often cytoreductive therapy, as hydroxyurea will help to slow the bone marrow proliferation and AVWS.

Usually, cytoreductive treatment is not immediately effective and additional treatments can be required in active bleeding patients [16].

Use of aspirin is recommended in PV and ET, nevertheless, the use of aspirin should be held until the cytoreductive therapy has lowered the platelet count to $<1000 \times 10^9/L$ [16].

5. Conclusions

The importance of early suspicion and diagnosis of AVWS remains on the clinical significance that major bleeding has in mortality and morbidity in patients regarding the underlying disease.

A non-family history of bleeding related to an underlying disease is the first aspect to consider for the diagnosis of AVWS.

In myeloproliferative neoplasms, AVWS would present with platelet counts above $500 \times 10^9/L$.

According to the guidelines, patients with ET who present with platelet counts greater than $1000 \times 10^9/L$ should be screened for AVWS. A VWF: Gplb or VWF: RCo/ VWF: Ag ratio < 0.7 in MPN would suggest AVWS.

Otherwise, we also suggest screening for AVWS in patients with PV, even though screening is not included in international guidelines for PV. Our statement is based on the recent findings that patients with AVWS and PV could present an elevated hematocrit associated with higher shear stress regardless of the platelet counts.

Although JAK2 V617F is the most common gene driver mutation found in myeloproliferative neoplasms, 95% of PV cases are related to this mutation.

Also, it is the most associated with a high-risk thrombosis profile and the most frequently found in AVWS.

Treatment of AVWS in MPN is based on multifactorial therapy, including treatment of underlying disease that would reverse AVWS.

Acknowledgements

Special thanks to Anal. Biochem. Olga Veronica Barrales Benitez, Hilda Elizeth Hernández Juárez, Darinel Hernández Hernández, María del Rosario Villa Márquez.

Conflict of interest

The authors declare no conflict of interest.

Appendixes and nomenclature

ADAMTS13	Desintegrin-like and metalloprotease with thrombospondin type 1 motif no.13
aPTT	activated partial thromboplastin time
CALR	calreticulin
CBC	complete blood count
dDAVP	desmopressin
ET	essential thrombocythemia
ECMO	extracorporeal membrane oxygenation

ISTH	International Society on Thrombosis and Haemostasis
Gplb	glucoprotein 1
JAK2 V617F	Janus kinase 2
IVIG	intravenous immunoglobulin
MGUS	monoclonal gammopathy of undetermined significance
MPL	myeloproliferative leukemia protein (thrombopoietin receptor)
MPN	myeloproliferative neoplasms
PT	prothrombin time
rVIIa	recombinant factor VIIa
rVWF	recombinant von Willebrand Factor
VWD	von Willebrand disease
VWF	von Willebrand factor
VWF:RCo/VWF Ag	VWF: Ristocetin Cofactor/VWF Antigen ratio
VWF CB/VWF Ag	VWF: Collagen Binding/VWF Antigen

Author details

Mariem Pulido Flores, Ángel Gabriel Vargas Ruiz, Oscar Jaime Moreno García and Elena Tuna Aguilar*
Instituto Nacional de Ciencias Médicas y Nutrición Salvador Zubirán, Ciudad de México, México

*Address all correspondence to: elenatuna@yahoo.fr

References

[1] Song I-C, Kang S, Lee M-W, et al. Acquired von Willebrand syndrome in patients with Philadelphia-negative myeloproliferative neoplasm. Blood Research. 2023;**58**:42-50. DOI: 10.5045/br.2023.2022218

[2] Simone JV, Cornet JA, Abildgaard CF. Acquired von Willebrand's syndrome in systemic lupus erythematosus. Blood. 1968;**31**(6):806-812

[3] Rottenstreich A, Kleinstern G, Krichevsky S, Varon D, Lavie D, Kalish Y. Factors related to the development of acquired von Willebrand syndrome in patients with essential thrombocythemia and polycythemia vera. European Journal of Internal Medicine. 2017;**41**:49-54. DOI: 10.1016/j.ejim.2016.11.011

[4] Onimoe G, Grooms L, Perdue K, Ruymann F. Acquired von Willebrand syndrome in congenital heart disease: Does it promote an increased bleeding risk? British Journal of Haematology. 2011;**155**(5):622-624. DOI: 10.1111/j.1365-2141.2011.08732.x

[5] Federici AB, Budde U, Castaman G, Rand JH, Tiede A. Current diagnostic and therapeutic approaches to patients with acquired von Willebrand syndrome: A 2013 update. Seminars in Thrombosis and Hemostasis. 2013;**39**(2):191-201

[6] Federici AB. Acquired von Willebrand syndrome: An underdiagnosed and misdiagnosed bleeding complication in patients with lymphoproliferative and myeloproliferative disorders. Seminars in Hematology. 2006;**43**(1 Suppl. 1):S48-S58. DOI: 10.1053/j.seminhematol.2005.11.003

[7] Lancellotti S, Dragani A, Ranalli P, et al. Qualitative and quantitative modifications of von Willebrand factor in patients with essential thrombocythemia and controlled platelet count. Journal of Thrombosis and Haemostasis. 2015;**13**:1226-1237

[8] Franchini M, Mannucci PM. Acquired von Willebrand syndrome: Focused for hematologists. Haematologica. 2020;**105**(8):2032-2037. DOI: 10.3324/haematol.2020.255117

[9] Mannucci PM. New therapies for von Willebrand disease. Blood Advances. 2019;**3**(21):3481-3487. DOI: 10.1182/bloodadvances.2019000368

[10] Franchini M, Manucci PM. Von Willebrand disease-associated angiodysplasia: A few answers, still many questions. British Journal of Haematology. 2013;**161**(2):177-182. DOI: 10.1111/bjh.12272

[11] Collins P, Budde U, Rand JH, Federici AB, Kessler CM. Epidemiology and general guidelines of the management of acquired haemophilia and von Willebrand syndrome. Haemophilia. 2008;**14**(Suppl. 3):49-55. DOI: 10.1111/j.1365-2516.2008.01745.x

[12] Tefferi A, Hanson CA, Kurtin PJ, Katzmann JA, Dalton RJ, Nichols WL. Acquired von Willebrand's disease due to aberrant expression of platelet glycoprotein Ib by marginal zone lymphoma cells. British Journal of Haematology. 1997;**96**(4):850-853. DOI: 10.1046/j.1365-2141.1997.d01-2088.x

[13] Scrobohaci ML, Daniel MT, Levy Y, Marolleau JP, Brouet JC. Expression of GpIb on plasma cells in a patient with monoclonal IgG and acquired von Willebrand disease. British Journal

of Haematology. 1993;**84**(3):471-475. DOI: 10.1111/j.1365-2141.1993.tb03103.x

[14] Shim K, Anderson PJ, Tuley EA, Wiswall E, Sadler JE. Platelet-VWF complexes are preferred substrates of ADAMTS13 under fluid shear stress. Blood. 2008;**111**:651-657

[15] Raife TJ, Cao W, Atkinson BS, et al. Leukocyte proteases cleave von Willebrand factor at or near the ADAMTS13 cleavage site. Blood. 2009;**114**:1666-1674

[16] Tiede A, Rand JH, Budde U, Ganser A, Federici AB. How I treat the acquired von Willebrand syndrome. Blood. 2011;**117**(25):6777-6785. DOI: 10.1182/blood-2010-11297580

[17] Tefferi A, Barbui T. Personalized management of essential thrombocythemia-application of recent evidence to clinical practice. Leukemia. 2013;**27**:1617-1620

[18] Tefferi A. Polycythemia vera and essential thrombocythemia: 2015 update on diagnosis, risk-stratification, and management. American Journal of Hematology. 2015;**90**:162-173

[19] Federici AB, Rand JH, Bucciarelli P, et al. Acquired von Willebrand syndrome: Data from an international registry. Thrombosis and Haemostasis. 2000;**84**(2):345-349

[20] Federici AB, Stabile F, Castaman G, Canciani MT, Mannucci PM. Treatment of acquired von Willebrand syndrome in patients with monoclonal gammopathy of uncertain significance: Comparison of three different therapeutic approaches. Blood. 1998;**92**:2707-2711

[21] Friederich PW, Wever PC, Briet E, Doorenbos CJ, Levi M. Successful treatment with recombinant factor VIIa of therapy-resistant severe bleeding in a patient with acquired von Willebrand disease. American Journal of Hematology. 2001;**66**:292-294

Chapter 2

Role of Anti-Prothrombin and Anti-Phosphatidylserine Antibodies in Altering Clotting Times

Antonio Ciampa and Mariachiara Gagliardi

Abstract

Anti-phospholipid syndrome (APS) is an autoimmune disease characterized by the presence of anti-phospholipid antibodies (aPL) in serum/plasma along with clinical manifestations such as thrombosis (both arterial and venous), fetal losses, hemolytic anemia, and thrombocytopenia. The laboratory signs of APS are persistent positivity of lupus anticoagulant (LA) and/or anticardiolipin antibodies (aCL) and/or anti-β2-glycoprotein I antibodies (β2-GPI). For other laboratory tests, such as prothrombin antibodies (aPT) or anti-phosphatidylserine antibodies (aPS), further standardization and/or studies are considered necessary to demonstrate an actual correlation with the clinical symptoms of the syndrome. This condition is particularly important in the determination of aPS/prothrombin time (PT). In this chapter, studies on the role of aPT/aPS in APS are summarized and discussed, and a literature review is presented, followed by a more detailed description of phosphatidylserine and human prothrombin; the detection of aPT and aPS/PT and the mechanisms causing the clinical event are described. Finally, a clinical case with a strange, prolonged activated partial thromboplastin time (aPTT) is presented, in which aPS/PT was a risk factor for the patient's life.

Keywords: anti-phospholipid syndrome (APS), anti-prothrombin antibodies (aPT), lupus anticoagulant (LA), anti-phosphatidylserine antibodies (aPS), activated partial thromboplastin time (aPTT)

1. Introduction

Anti-phospholipid antibodies (aPL) are a heterogeneous family of antibodies/immunoglobulins directed against various compounds such as negatively charged phospholipids (PL), plasma proteins, proteins of the membrane of endothelial cells, or platelets, with which they can form complexes due to their high affinity for anionic PL surfaces. The main antigens they target are β2-glycoprotein I (β2GPI), cardiolipin (CL), prothrombin (PT), phosphatidylserine (PS), annexin A5, annexin

A2, protein C, protein S, low-density oxidized lipoproteins, lysophosphatidic acid, and sulfatides. The most commonly used laboratory tests are the lupus anticoagulant (LA), the anticardiolipin antibodies (aCL), and the anti-β2 antibodies GPI (aβ2 GPI). For other antibody classes, such as the anti-prothrombin antibodies (aPT) and the anti-phosphatidylserine antibodies (aPS) or anti-phosphatidylserine-prothrombin antibodies (aPS/PT), it is not clear what role they play in APS. This situation is further complicated by the fact that the tests used to determine them need to be more standardized [1, 2]. There are hundreds of publications on this topic. The discussion of the literature mentioned follows.

2. Literature analysis

The literature shows that the assessment of aPS/PT in APS could help to define patients at high risk of clinical events (both thrombotic and hemorrhagic). In a multicenter international study, aPS/PT+, particularly the IgG isotype, were found to be markers for the presence of LA and were also strongly associated with the presence of clinical events related to APS [3]. A recent prospective study included 180 patients (with a follow-up of ±31 months) in which aPS/PT was assessed in addition to the aPLs included in the Sydney APS criteria (aCL and aβ2 GPI). The highest incidence of thrombosis was found in aPS/PT+ patients with LA+/aCL+/aβ2GPI+ compared to patients with triple or double positivity [4]. Some research groups have proposed quantifying the risk of clinical events in APS using an aPL score (aPL-S). The work involves multiple assessments of aPLs (LA/aCL/aβ2GPI/aPS/PT) and assigning a specific clinical value to each essay and its title [5]. There is also another score called GAPSS (global APS score) that takes into account the aPL profile (LA/aCL/aβ2GPI/aPS/PT) and classic cardiovascular risk factors [6]. The association with the clinical features of APS has been shown to increase correlatively with these scores (which include evidence of aPS/PT). For this reason, assessment of aPS/PT would be a very useful quantitative marker in APS. A review by Sciascia et al. analyzed Medline publications between 1988 and 2013 examining aPT and aPS/PT as a risk factor for thrombosis. Whenever possible, antibody isotypes and sites of thrombosis were analyzed. Antibodies to PT (both aPT and aPS/PT) have a higher risk of thrombosis (OR 2.3; 95% CI: 1.7–3.5). aPS/PT antibodies appeared to be a stronger risk factor for thrombosis than aPT, both for arterial and venous thrombosis (OR 5.1; 95% CI: 4.2–6.3 and OR 1.8; 95% CI: 1.4–2.7, respectively). In conclusion, routine measurement of aPS/PT (but not aPT) may be useful to determine the risk of thrombosis in patients with previous thrombosis and/or systemic lupus erythematosus (SLE) [7]. In a paper published by Forastiero et al. in 2005, the thrombotic risk of aβ2GPI and aPT antibodies was investigated in a cohort of 194 consecutive patients with persistent LA and/or aCL. The average follow-up period was 45 months. A total of 39 patients (20%) had a documented thrombosis during follow-up. Eleven of these patients had no thrombosis before entering the study and 28 had recurrences. There were 21 venous and 18 arterial thrombotic events and the overall incidence of thrombosis was 5.6% per patient per year. Patients who were positive for aβ2GPI thus had a higher rate of thrombosis than patients with aPL without aβ2GPI (8.0% vs. 3.1% per patient/year). Similarly, a higher thrombosis rate was found in patients with aPT compared to patients without aPT (8.6% vs. 3.5% per patient/year). Considering only the group of 142 patients with positive LA, the highest incidence of thrombosis was found in patients with LA for both aβ2GPI and aPT (8.4% per patient/year) [8]. In 2000,

Atsumi published the results of a study of 265 patients attending the Autoimmune Disease Clinic. The presence of aPS/PT, but not aPT, was significantly correlated with the clinical manifestations of APS (OR 4.4), and aPS/PT were as specific as aCL and aβ2GPI. IgG aPS/PT was strongly correlated with the presence of LA with dRVVT+ (OR 38.2) [9]. For their part, Zhang et al. examined a total of 441 subjects, including 101 patients with primary APS (PAPS), 140 with secondary APS (SAPS), 161 disease controls (DC), and 39 healthy controls (HC). APS/PT IgG/IgM levels were significantly higher in patients with APS compared to DC and HC. aPS/PT-IgG and IgM were present in 29.7% and 54.5% of PAPS and 42.1% and 53.6% of SAPS, respectively. LA had the highest OR (3.6) in identifying patients with thrombosis, followed by aCL-IgG (OR 2.6), aPS/PT-IgG (OR 2.5), and aβ2GPI1 IgG (OR 2.3) [10]. In 2017, Shi et al. published a study of the prevalence and clinical associations of aPS/PT with thrombosis and pregnancy loss in Chinese patients with APS and seronegative APS (APS-SN). One hundred eighty-six patients with APS, 48 with APS-SN, 176 disease controls, 79 SLE, 29 Sjögren's syndrome, 30 ankylosing spondylitis, 38 rheumatoid arthritis, and 90 healthy donors were studied. One hundred sixty (86%) of the APS patients were positive for at least one aPS/PT isotype. One hundred thirty-five (72%) were positive for aPS/PT-IgG, 124 (66%) for aPS/PT-IgM, and 99 (53%) for both [11]. Approximately half of the APS-SN patients were positive for aPS/PT-IgG and/or IgM. Highly significant associations were found between aPS/PT-IgG and venous thrombotic events (OR 6.7) and aPS/PT IgG/IgM and pregnancy loss (OR 9.4). Two further research studies investigated the relationship between aPS/PT and complications during pregnancy. The studies found that aPS/PT is associated with severe blood clotting, severe pregnancy problems leading to preterm delivery, and small vessel disease, all of which occur in high-risk cases of APS and require intensive treatment [12–14]. Occasionally, aPL coagulopathy may begin with a hemorrhagic syndrome in the presence of severe thrombocytopenia, acquired thrombocytopathy, acquired factor VIII inhibitor, or acquired prothrombin deficiency. Typically, APL-related thrombocytopenia is mild and shows no clinical symptoms. Bleeding rarely occurs in patients with APS, except in certain cases, for example, when thrombocytopenia is associated with thrombotic microangiopathy, as is the case in catastrophic APS. If the platelet count falls below 30×10^9/L and bleeding symptoms occur, the same treatments are given for idiopathic thrombocytopenic purpura. Sometimes, a bleeding disorder caused by non-neutralizing anti-prothrombin antibodies can occur, leading to severe hypoprothrombinemia. The primary effects of APS are thrombosis and pregnancy loss. However, there are other clinical symptoms associated with the presence of persistent autoimmune APS. Bleeding is rare but may be the first sign in individuals with severe thrombocytopenia or prothrombin deficiency [15]. Based on the clinical evidence collected in the literature, it is likely that aPS/PT will be included in the new criteria for the diagnosis of APS in the future.

3. What are phosphatidylserine and prothrombin?

3.1 Phosphatidylserine

As we already know, numerous plasma proteins, known as factors and cofactors, are involved in the coagulation mechanism. This enzymatic chain process leads to a progressive amplification of the original signal. PLs play a crucial role by providing an anchoring surface that facilitates the interaction between the different components of the coagulation cascade. Vitamin K-dependent factors (PT and factors VII, IX, and X) bind to phospholipid surfaces via their γ-carboxyglutamic acid residues (Gla domains) in the presence of calcium ions. The binding of calcium to the Gla residues leads to a conformational change that exposes the hydrophobic sites necessary for protein binding. Factors V and VIII (cofactors), PT, and thrombin-activated factor X bind to phospholipid membranes to form the respective activation complexes of FX to FXa and PT to thrombin. The speed of the coagulation process depends on the chemical composition of the PL and the properties of the phospholipid membrane surface. Biological lipid membranes are functionally and structurally asymmetric with large differences between the inner and outer layers. In most unstimulated cells, the PLs of the phosphatidylcholine (PC) and sphingomyelin type are located in the outer layer and PS, phosphatidylinositol (PI) and phosphatidylethanolamine (PE) in the inner layer. When the membranes are activated, the asymmetry is lost and PS, an anionic phospholipid, is exposed in the outer layer of the membrane. This exposure to an increased concentration of anionic phospholipid (PL) in the outer layer is essential for accelerating the activation reactions of the coagulation system. PS is the strongest and most efficient anionic PL responsible for this acceleration (**Figure 1**).

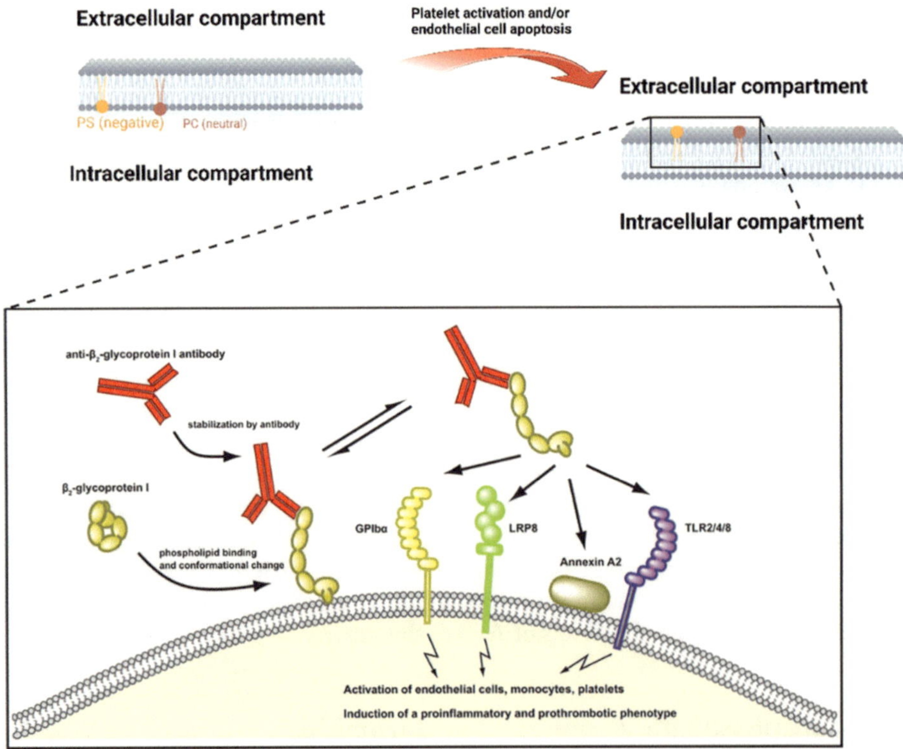

Figure 1.
The cell membrane consists of neutral PL (PC) and negatively charged PL (PS) that migrate to the outer layer during platelet and endothelial cell activation or apoptosis. β2GPI is not recognized by pathological anti-β2GPI antibodies in the circulation. When phospholipids are negatively charged, they are exposed and β2GPI binds to this surface and changes its conformation. This step exposes a cryptic epitope in domain I, which is recognized by the pathological antibodies. The antibody fixes β2GPI in this conformation, and the antibody-β2GPI complex can subsequently interact with various surface receptors, such as glycoprotein Ibα (GPIbα), LRP8, annexin A2 and several members of the TLR family (TLR2, -4 and -8) [16].

3.2 Human prothrombin

PT is an important antigenic target for aPL in APS. It is a 72 kDa, vitamin K-dependent, single-chain glycoprotein with three carbohydrate chains and 10 Gla domains. It circulates in normal plasma at an approximate concentration of 100 mg/mL. It is converted to thrombin in vivo by the action of the prothrombinase complex (FXa-FVa phospholipids and calcium ions) and in vitro by the presence of thromboplastin and calcium ions, which interact with plasma factors during the coagulation process. This activation reaction continues with the polymerization of fibrinogen to fibrin. It is one of the most important PL-binding proteins and was described as a cofactor of LA in 1959 [17]. The first data indicating that LA interferes at the level of the prothrombinase complex date back to 1965 [18]. In 1980, Xourgia et al. demonstrated for the first time that a monoclonal immunoglobulin M (IgM) with LA activity can block the binding of prothrombin and FX to phospholipid micelles [19]. In 1983, the first data were presented on the existence of antibodies with high affinity for PT, which were responsible for the formation of complexes that were rapidly eliminated from the bloodstream [17]. These antibodies were studied by immunodiffusion and characterized as non-neutralizing, as they did not react with the functional site of the protein. Later, cross-linked immunoelectrophoresis studies showed that aPT complexes were also present in patients with normal PT levels [20]. The conclusion from these studies was that there are low-affinity antibodies that do not induce hypoprothrombinemia but are responsible for LA activity. The hypothesis was that the antibodies are polyreactive and react with epitopes located in the PL and PT [1]. These studies were performed with purified lgM from a patient with macroglobulinemia using immunodiffusion assays and showed that the antibody reacted specifically with anionic PL (PS and PI) and not with neutral PL (PE and PC). Similar results were obtained with immunoglobulin G (IgG) fractions purified by adsorption with LC liposomes and affinity column chromatography [21–23]. These experiments allowed us to postulate that the mechanism of action of aPL is to inhibit the binding of vitamin K-dependent factors to phospholipid surfaces. The type of PL present in membranes is important because PS has been shown to induce a profound conformational change in the PT molecule [24]. In a recent study, 18% of purified IgG with LA activity was found to be able to inhibit prothrombinase activity on endothelial cells. Other authors working with purified IgG postulated that LA binds to an epitope on the PT and then to the PL via a calcium-mediated PL-PT interaction. The results from these studies lead to the conclusion that LA exerts its anticoagulant effect and interaction with complement via calcium ions of the human PT with PL [25].

4. aPT and aPS/PT detection

There are two methods to identify antibodies directed against PT. They can be detected directly by ELISA with prothrombin-coated plates (to detect aPT) or using the phosphatidylserine/prothrombin complex as antigen (to detect aPS/PT). They are frequently found in patients with systemic lupus erythematosus (SLE) and their presence is associated with thrombosis. It should be noted that the prevalence of aPT in patients with APS varies greatly depending on the test used. In a 2002 retrospective review study conducted by Galli's group, 48% of patients with APS-related features who were negative on conventional tests had aPT antibodies, making these antibodies potential markers for APS [2]. Despite the association found between aPT and aPS/PT in APS, it appears that each of these antibodies belongs to a different group of antibodies. Recent studies have reported that the presence of aPT is not associated with a higher risk of thrombosis. However, a positive association between aPS/PT and the development of a procoagulant state has recently been observed, as they have been shown to have higher sensitivity and specificity than aCL with a significant correlation with LA and therefore could be potential candidates for a screening laboratory for the diagnosis of APS. There are commercial ELISA tests for the detection of aPS/PT. β2 GPI or apolipoprotein H is the antigen most relevant to the disease. In 1990, various studies showed that this protein is necessary for the binding of aCL to PL and acts as a "cofactor." Negatively charged PL antibodies include IgG and IgM isotypes that can be directed against CL, PI, PS, phosphatidic acid (PA), PE, lysobisphosphatidic acid (LBPA), and sulfatides. The diagnostic and prognostic value of these antibodies has been calculated, and it has been found that, apart from aCL, the antibodies against PS are the most important. However, the evaluation of these antibodies does not increase the probability of diagnosis, so their clinical use is not currently justified. In research studies, antibodies against PS and PE have been associated with obstetric complications [1, 26, 27].

5. Proposed mechanisms of aPL-mediated thrombosis

The understanding of the pathophysiology of the disease has made great progress since the 1990s thanks to animal models (immunization of mice with aPL) and the knowledge of the interaction between aPL and various components of blood coagulation and the endothelium. It has also been shown that inflammation plays an important role in the development of the disease [28]. A proposed mechanism to explain aPL-mediated thrombosis would be as follows: the cell membrane is composed of neutral PL (PC) and negatively charged PL (PS), which migrate to the outer layer during platelet and endothelial cell activation or apoptosis. Dimeric β2 GPI normally binds to PS via receptors such as annexin A2 or Toll-like receptors (TLR), inhibiting the activation of the coagulation cascade on endothelial cells. aPL binds to β2 GPI, interfering with its function and activating the complement system by inducing the expression of C5a, which in turn triggers the expression of adhesion molecules, cytokines, and tissue factor (TF). Monocytes are also activated by protease receptors, polymorphonuclear (PMN), which form networks of DNA and platelets, leading to the release of proinflammatory mediators and the generation of a prothrombotic state. Moreover, it is now known that p38 mitogen-activated protein kinase (p38-MAPK) (a fundamental protein for the cellular response to stress) and nuclear factor kB (NF-kB, a fundamental transcription factor in inflammatory processes, activation, proliferation, etc.) play an important role in the cascade of intracellular signals leading to platelet activation and adhesion, increased TF expression and cytokine release (**Figure 1**) [25, 28, 29]. In the case of aPTs, the mechanisms underlying the procoagulant properties are not known. Two possibilities are currently postulated: (a) by humoral regulators of coagulation (PT) or (b) by activation/deactivation of cellular receptors. One anecdotal report suggests that polyclonal antibodies from patients with aPT may act on a "target molecule" expressed on the surface of endothelial cells, although this has not yet been characterized. It has been reported that aPS/PT-induced TF production in procoagulant cells occurs predominantly via activation of the p38 MAPK signaling pathway, like the mechanisms involved in aβ2 GPI-induced cell activation. In mice, active immunization with PT is associated with increased thrombosis, arguing for the role of aPT in thrombus formation. In addition, mice treated with IS6 (a murine aPT monoclonal antibody) show thrombi that are larger and persist longer than in mice injected with the control antibody [27].

6. Role of aPS/PT in the diagnosis of APS

In clinical practice, the determination of aCL, β2 GPI and LA are currently the tests defined in the Sydney Consensus for the diagnosis of APS. The clinical relevance of other aPL tests for antibodies other than those mentioned is currently under discussion. Numerous studies have been conducted to demonstrate their usefulness for the diagnosis of APS in patients with thrombosis and/or pregnancy morbidity, particularly in patients who are repeatedly negative on the 2006 criteria tests. Among the non-conventional aPL tests, aPS/PT has been proposed as a potential marker to assess thrombosis risk and pregnancy morbidity in patients with suspected APS. The positivity profile is key to defining clinical risk and increases in parallel with the titer and combination of aPL. The risk of thrombotic events increases progressively with the number of positive aPL determinations [17]. The highest risk of thrombosis, thromboembolic recurrence, and obstetric complications is associated with triple positivity for aPL. It was found that aPS/PT, in combination with LA and aβ2 GPI, identified the highest risk group for APS in patients with SLE. The role of aPT, aPS/PT, anti-annexin A5, aPC, and aPS antibodies in APS remains to be defined. As already mentioned, the relationship between aPL and thromboembolic events is extensive and well-documented. However, acquired coagulopathy caused by aPL is complex and can occasionally manifest as a hemorrhagic event with varying clinical severity or as a combined thrombo-hemorrhagic syndrome. The latter often occurs in catastrophic APS (CAPS), a rare but often fatal variant with excessive activation of hemostasis, consumption of its components, and micro-thrombotic damage in multiple organs. aPL can interact with various blood and vascular components and cause bleeding via several mechanisms. First, aPL-positive patients often develop thrombocytopenia. Second, acquired immune-mediated coagulation factor deficiencies such as hypoprothrombinemia can occur as a result of the interaction between aPL and coagulation factors. Thirdly, damage to the microvascular system due to an extensive thrombotic or inflammatory insult can lead to secondary bleeding in the affected tissue via the activation of monocytes, endothelial cells, and complement (**Figure 1**). Thrombotic microangiopathies (TMAs) such as CAPS as well as diffuse alveolar hemorrhage (DAH) and adrenal hemorrhage (AH), the pathognomonic complications of APS, are representative examples of this pathomechanism [18]. As antithrombotic therapy remains a mainstay of treatment for APS, the extensive use of antithrombotics typical of affected patients can contribute to bleeding and is the fourth cause. Severe thrombocytopenia (platelet count below 50,000/μL) and prothrombin deficiency are the most important causes of bleeding. The discussion of the pathomechanisms mentioned follows.

7. Factor deficiencies associated with aPL

7.1 Hypoprothrombinemia

Acquired prothrombin deficiency, also known as lupus anticoagulant hypoprothrombinemia syndrome, is the best-known and best-defined of all coagulation factor deficiencies associated with aPL. The exact incidence is unclear, but with an order of magnitude of hundreds of reported cases, it appears to be a rare complication [30, 31]. It typically occurs in pediatric or adolescent patients with aPL after viral infections or in systemic immune diseases, most commonly in SLE [32]. Adults can also be affected, although less frequently [23, 33]. Pre-existing systemic immune disease is not essential, as cases without this condition have also been reported. Other triggering conditions include tumors such as lymphomas, especially with the production of pathological immunoglobulins and drug reactions. The severity of bleeding varies from mild mucocutaneous bleeding (epistaxis, ecchymosis), which is the most common, to severe and life-threatening bleeding, which also affects localizations such as muscles, genitourinary tract, gastrointestinal tract (GIT), and central nervous system (CNS) [34–37]. A considerable number of patients (up to 50%) do not experience significant bleeding and may even be asymptomatic [17]. The simultaneous occurrence of thrombotic events, hemorrhagic-thrombotic syndrome, and CAPS has occasionally been described [38–40]. The disease is usually self-limiting when associated with viral infections, whereas in autoimmune diseases it may be of long duration or occur in episodes [17]. Despite the possibility of severe bleeding, the overall prognosis is generally good, with a reported mortality rate of less than 5%. Laboratory findings include prolonged prothrombin time (PT) and activated partial thromboplastin time (aPTT), variably decreased prothrombin activity (on average about 10–20%, although it can also be extremely low or unmeasurable) with a proportional decrease in prothrombin antigen. As already mentioned, there may also be a deficiency of other coagulation factors. Their activity should therefore be checked [30]. A positive test for LA completes the picture. The finding of PT prolongation in an aPL-positive patient should prompt testing for prothrombin deficiency, even if no bleeding is evident at this time [18]. The traditional view, based on the first analyses in the 1980s, defines the antibodies involved as non-neutralizing, that is, they are not able to directly inhibit the coagulation activity of prothrombin [4]. A probable explanation is the cross-reactivity between the aPL and the phospholipid epitopes in the prothrombin molecules: the aPL form prothrombin-antigen-antibody complexes, and their subsequent elimination leads to a proportional decrease in both prothrombin activity and antigen. If clearance is extensive enough to lead to a relevant decrease in prothrombin with activity below 20%, bleeding manifestations may occur. However, some researchers have presented conflicting evidence suggesting more complex changes in hemostasis. In the most recent analysis of a relatively large cohort of 41 patients, the Japanese authors were unable to establish a precise correlation between prothrombin levels, anti-FII antibody levels, and bleeding phenotype. In addition to anti-prothrombin antibodies, they also identified various autoantibodies directed against FVIII in several patients with the disease [41]. A small number of the cases examined also confirmed combined coagulation factor deficiencies. Based on this observation and the known heterogeneity of the clinical presentation, it can be concluded that hypoprothrombinaemia is not an isolated alteration in aPL-positive patients and always requires a complex evaluation of hemostasis. The therapeutic approach aims to (1) stop the active bleeding, (2) eliminate the antibodies responsible for the prothrombin deficiency, and (3) prevent further thromboembolic events [35, 36]. Discontinuation of antithrombotic drugs, supplementation of blood components (transfusion of packed red blood cells and fresh frozen plasma), activation of clotting factor production (administration of vitamin K), hemostatic agents (styptics, antifibrinolytics) are the strategies to stop bleeding [34, 42]. However, all of these approaches can lead to an increased risk of thrombosis in aPL-positive patients, especially with prolonged use. Immunosuppression with corticosteroids as the first choice or other agents (azathioprine, rituximab, cyclophosphamide) and procedures (plasma exchange) as alternatives leads to eradication of the antibodies. Monotherapy with corticosteroids is effective in most cases. Measurement of prothrombin levels, whether by coagulation, chromogenic or immunologic methods, can be used to monitor treatment. Since the risk of thrombosis generally remains significantly increased even in the presence of bleeding and bleeding itself does not protect against thromboembolism, therapies aimed at stopping bleeding must be balanced by antithrombotic therapy. Both the risk of bleeding and the risk of thromboembolism must be carefully weighed up in each individual case.

7.2 Von Willebrand factor deficiency (von Willebrand syndrome) and deficiencies of other coagulation factors

There are few case reports of the concomitant presence of acquired von Willebrand syndrome (AWS), acquired vWF deficiency, and the presence of aPL [41, 43–46]. Interestingly, other diseases with a clearly defined relationship to AWS (myeloproliferative neoplasms, aortic valve stenosis, and connective tissue diseases such as SLE) were found in most cases [44]. Therefore, aPL is not considered a common cause of AWS but rather an incidental finding in underlying immune disorders. Some researchers have speculated that aPL may modify and compensate for the bleeding phenotype typical of AWS [41, 46]. A thrombotic event has been reported after normalization of vWF levels [41]. Immunosuppression, the standard treatment of AWS, in combination with antithrombotic prophylaxis, was performed in the reported cases with good clinical results. Acquired deficiencies of other coagulation factors, namely FVII, FVIII, FX, and FXI, have been reported [47, 48]. In summary, these deficiencies are extremely rare and clinical data are limited to case reports. The bleeding manifestations are variable and of varying severity. The therapeutic strategies are similar to the approach used in AWS.

8. How aPS/PT can alter aPTT: A case report

8.1 Case report

A 46-year-old female patient with no previous illnesses was diagnosed with a meningioma. As the meningioma was to be removed, the patient underwent a routine preoperative examination. The laboratory examination revealed a high aPTT ratio (2.11; reference range 0.85–1.20) with a normal prothrombin time (PT) ratio (1.05; reference range 0.80–1.15). In order to understand the causes for the prolongation of the aPTT ratio, further investigations were carried out. The mixing test (in which the patient's plasma was mixed with a pool of normal plasma in a 1:1 ratio) resulted in an aPTT ratio of 1.12, which is why a factor deficiency was initially assumed. However, the coagulation factors were all normal (**Table 1**). A dRVVT (diluted Russell's viper venom time) was then performed to look for the LA, but this was also negative (dRVVT screening ratio 0.85). As a bleeding disorder was feared, a bleeding time measurement was performed, which confirmed that the patient was unable to coagulate within the indicated times (reference range < 5 minutes). Since bleeding time evaluates the vascular and thrombocytic phase of hemostasis, a platelet function test was also performed, but it was normal. Finally, another test was performed to look for LA: The silica clotting time (SCT). This differs from the dRVVT due to the different concentrations of the phospholipid mixture. The patient's SCT-normal ratio was 2.45 (reference range < 1.20). This meant that the patient had non-specific inhibitors that caused prolongation of the aPTT. Tests for aCL and aB2GPI IgG/IgM were performed, which were negative. A search was then performed for aPS/PT IgG/IgM. The patient had high titers of aPS/PT class IgG (all test data are listed in **Table 1**). Once the cause of the aPTT prolongation was known, the patient was prepared for removal of the meningioma: The day before surgery and the same morning, the patient was treated with a drug containing coagulation factor VII: This drug induces blood coagulation at the site of the hemorrhage. This medication is used to treat bleeding and to prevent excessive bleeding after surgery or other major treatments. The operation was successful and without complications or bleeding episodes or thrombotic events.

8.2 Discussion

In relation to the case just presented, it must be emphasized that the hypoprothrombinemia associated with LAs is caused by anti-prothrombin (FII) antibodies,

Tests	Value	Reference range
PT	1.05	Ratio 0.80–1.15
aPTT	2.11	Ratio 0.85–1.20
aPTT-mix	1.12	Ratio 0.85–1.20
Fibrinogen	124	<250 μg/dL
Platelet	215	$\times 10^9$/L
Bleeding time	11	<5 minutes
Factor II	87	79–131%
Factor V	99	62–139%
Factor VII	102	50–120%
Factor VIII	97	50–150%
Factor IX	95	65–150%
Factor X	101	77–131%
Factor XI	94	65–150%
Factor XII	112	50–150%
Von Willebrand factor	124	O 41–125% A, B, AB 61–157%
LA: dRVVT	0.85	Normalized ratio < 1.20
LA: SCT	2.45	Normalized ratio < 1.25
β2GPI-IgG	7.2	<20 Unit/mL
β2GPI-IgM	4.9	<20 Unit/mL
aCL-IgG	8.3	<20 Unit/mL
aCL-IgM	6.1	<20 Unit/mL
aPS/PT-IgG	86.4	<20 Unit/mL
aPS/PT-IgM	23.2	<20 Unit/mL

Table 1.
All data regarding the tests performed on the patient are listed in the table.

which are heterogeneous and may be directed against prothrombin or the phosphatidylserine/prothrombin complex. They usually act by a "non-neutralizing" mechanism that increases the clearance of the antibody factor. They are diagnosed by a positive lupus anticoagulant test, prolonged activated partial thromboplastin time (aPTT), low FII levels, positive inhibitor screening (mix test) and detection of an anti-prothrombin antibody. In this case, there was a number of data that did not fit the above profile and raised many questions among laboratory technicians and clinicians. The patient had a completely normal aPTT mixing time, FII ratio, and dRVVT ratio. This emphasizes that in some cases, it is necessary to perform different tests to look for LA: DRVVT, unlike SCT, was not able to detect the presence of inhibitors. Moreover, in some cases, the aPTT mixture may be normal even in the presence of inhibitors, especially if it is the aPS/PT type. In summary, this case should give us pause for thought as to whether there is still no standardized diagnostic procedure for the detection of aPT/PS. But given the clinical relevance of aPT/PS, further efforts should be made to create an effective diagnostic pathway.

9. Conclusion and future

In summary, anti-prothrombin antibodies (aPT and/or aPS/PT) are frequently found in patients with anti-phospholipid antibodies. Their immunological and functional properties are highly variable and depend mainly on their affinity to human prothrombin. Despite the increasing knowledge of their mechanisms of action, the clinical relevance of these antibodies is not yet clear. This is partly because their presence has also been identified in diseases other than anti-phospholipid syndrome. Future works should aim to determine whether these antibodies play a role in the pathogenesis of the common complications of anti-phospholipid syndrome. Bleeding is a rare but potentially serious complication of APS. The etiology is heterogeneous. APL-positive patients can develop bleeding due to thrombocytopenia, acquired coagulation factor deficiencies (predominantly hypoprothrombinemia), TMAs, or the adverse effects of antithrombotic therapy (usually with warfarin). However, thromboembolic events are the most dangerous complications for aPL-positive patients, and the risk of thrombosis remains clinically relevant even in the presence of bleeding in the majority of patients. In the future, aPL-positive patients receiving antithrombotics should be closely monitored and compliance ensured, especially in the scenario with high-intensity or combined antithrombotic therapy.

Conflict of interest

The authors declare no conflict of interest.

Appendixes and nomenclature

aCL	anticardiolipin antibodies
aPL	anti-phospholipid antibodies
aβ2GPI	anti-β2 glycoprotein I
aβ2GPI-D1	anti-β2 domain 1 glycoprotein I
APS	anti-phospholipid syndrome

aPT	anti-prothrombin
aPS/PT	anti-phosphatidylserine/prothrombin
aPS	anti-phosphatidylserine
aPL-S	aPL score
aGAPSS	adjusted global APS score
CL	cardiolipin
dRVVT	dilute Russell viper venom time
ELISA	enzyme-linked immuno sorbent assay
GAPSS	global APS score
Ig	immunoglobulin
LA	lupus anticoagulant
NF-kB	nuclear factor kB
OR	odds ratio
PS	phosphatidylserine
PA	phosphatidic acid
PT	prothrombin
PL	phospholipid
PC	phosphatidyl choline
RIA	radioimmunoassay
SCT	silica clotting time
SLE	systemic lupus erythematosus
SAPS	secondary anti-phospholipid syndrome

Author details

Antonio Ciampa* and Mariachiara Gagliardi
AORN San Giuseppe Moscati, Hemostasis Centre, Avellino, Italy

*Address all correspondence to: ciampa@inopera.it

References

[1] Misasi R, Capozzi A, Longo A, et al. "New" antigenic targets and methodological approaches for refining laboratory diagnosis of antiphospholipid syndrome. Journal of Immunology Research. 2015;**15**:1-13

[2] Galli M, Luciani D, Bertolini G, et al. Lupus anticoagulants are stronger risk factors for thrombosis than anticardiolipin antibodies in the antiphospholipid syndrome: A systematic review. Blood. 2003;**101**:1827-1832

[3] Amengual O, Foreigner R, Sugiura-Ogasawara M, et al. Evaluation of phosphatidylserine-dependent antiprothrombin antibody testing for the diagnosis of antiphospholipid syndrome: Results of an international multicentre study. Lupus. 2017;**26**:266-276

[4] Bajaj SP, Rapaport SI, Fierer DS, et al. A mechanism for the hypoprothrombinemia of the acquired hypoprothrombinemia lupus anticoagulant syndrome. Blood. 1983;**61**:684-692

[5] Yin ET, Gaston LW. Purification and kinetic studies on a circulating anticoagulant in a suspected case of lupus erythematosus. Thrombosis et Diathesis Haemorrhagica. 1965;**14**:88-95

[6] Thiagarajan P, Shapiro S, De Marco L. Monoclonal immunoglobulin M coagulation inhibitor with phospholipid specificity: Mechanism of a lupus anticoagulant. The Journal of Clinical Investigation. 1980;**66**:397-405

[7] Fleck RA, Rapaport SI, Rao LVM. Anti-prothrombin antibodies and the lupus anticoagulant. Blood. 1988;**72**:512-519

[8] Pengo V, Thiagarajan P, Shapiro SS, et al. Immunologic specificity and subgroups mechanism of action of IgG lupus anticoagulant. Blood. 1987;**70**:69-76

[9] Harris EN, Gharavi AE, Tincani A, et al. Affinity purified anti-cardiolipin antibodies and anti-DNA antibodies. Journal of Clinical & Laboratory Immunology. 1985;**17**:155-162

[10] Harris EN, Pierangeli S, Birch D. Anticardiolipin wet workshop report. Fifth International Symposium on antiphospholipid antibodies. American Journal of Clinical Pathology. 1994;**101**:616-624

[11] Shi H, Hui H, Yin YF, et al. Antiphosphatidylserine/prothrombin antibodies (aPS/PT) as potential diagnostic markers and risk predictors of venous thrombosis and obstetric complications in antiphospholipid syndrome. Clinical Chemistry and Laboratory Medicine (CCLM). 2018;**54**:614-619

[12] Wu JR, Lentz BR. Phospholipid-specific conformational changes in human prothrombin upon binding to procoagulant acidic lipid membranes. Thrombosis and Haemostasis. 1994;7:596-604

[13] Oosting JD, Derksen RHWM, Bobbink IWG, et al. Antiphospholipid antibodies directed against a combination of phospholipids with prothrombin, protein C or protein S: An explanation for their pathogenic mechanism? Blood. 1993;**81**:2618-2625

[14] Alessandri C, Conti F, Pendolino M, et al. New autoantigens in the antiphospholipid syndrome. Autoimmunity Reviews. 2011;**10**:609-616

[15] Forastiero R. Bleeding in the antiphospholipid syndrome. Hematology;**17**(sup1):153-155

[16] Misasi R, Longo A, Recalchi S, et al. Molecular mechanisms of “antiphospholipid antibodies” and their paradoxical role in the pathogenesis of “seronegative APS”. International Journal of Molecular Sciences. 2020;**21**:8411-8419

[17] Giannakopoulos B, Krilis SA. The pathogenesis of the antiphospholipid syndrome. The New England Journal of Medicine. 2013;**368**:1033-1039

[18] Kubisz P, Holly P, Stasko J. Bleeding in patients with antiphospholipid antibodies. In: Antiphospholipid Syndrome—Recent Advances in Clinical and Basic Aspects. London, UK: IntechOpen; 2022

[19] Xourgia E, Tektonidou MG. Management of non-criteria manifestations in antiphospholipid syndrome. Current Rheumatology Reports. 2020;**22**:1-13

[20] Alarcon-Segovia D, Perez-Vasquez ME, Villa AR, Drenkard C, Cabiedes J. Preliminary classification criteria for the antiphospholipid syndrome within systemic lupus erythematosus. Seminars in Arthritis and Rheumatism. 1992;**21**:275-286

[21] Andrews PA, Frampton G, Cameron JS. Antiphospholipid syndrome and systemic lupus erythematosus. Lancet. 1993;**342**:988-989

[22] Asherson RA. A "primary" antiphospholipid syndrome? The Journal of Rheumatology. 1988;**15**:1741-1746

[23] Asherson RA, Baguley E, Pal C, et al. Antiphospholipid syndrome: Five year follow up. Annals of the Rheumatic Diseases. 1991;**50**:805-810

[24] Asherson RA, Cervera R, Piette JC, et al. The Antiphospholipid Syndrome. Vol. 1. Boca Raton, FL: CRC Press; 1996. pp. 45-89

[25] Asherson RA, Khamashta MA, Ordi-Ros J, et al. The "primary" antiphospholipid syndrome: Major clinical and serological features. Medicine (Baltimore). 1989;**68**:366-374

[26] Blanco Y, Ramos-Casals M, Garcia-Carrasco M, et al. Sindrome antifosfolipidico primario que evoluciona a lupus eritematoso sistemico: Presentacion de tres nuevos casos y revision de la literatura. Revista Clínica Española. 1999;**199**:586-588

[27] Branch DW, Andres R, Digre KB, et al. The association of antiphospholipid antibodies with severe preeclampsia. Obstetrics and Gynecology. 1989;**73**:541-545

[28] Branch DW, Silver RM, Blackwell JL, et al. Outcome of treated pregnancies in women with antiphospholipid syndrome: An update of the Utah experience. Obstetrics and Gynecology. 1992;**80**:614-620

[29] Carbone J, Orera M, Rodriguez-Mahou M, et al. Immunological abnormalities in primary APS evolving into SLE: 6 years follow-up in women with repeated pregnancy loss. Lupus. 1999;**8**:274-278

[30] Gonzalez-Lopez TJ, Alvarez-Roman MT, Pascual C, et al. Use of eltrombopag for secondary immune thrombocytopenia in clinical practice. British Journal of Haematology. 2017;**178**:959-970

[31] Guitton Z, Terriou L, Lega JC, et al. Risk of thrombosis with antiphospholipid syndrome in systemic lupus erythematosus treated with

thrombopoietin receptor agonists. Rheumatology (Oxford, England). 2018;**57**:1432-1438

[32] Yu-Hin Chan E, Leung KFS, Soo ETL, et al. A Chinese boy with lupus anticoagulant-hypoprothrombinemia syndrome: A case report and review of the literature. Journal of Pediatric Hematology/Oncology. 2020;**13**:17-22

[33] LaMoreaux B, Barbar-Smiley F, Ardoin S, et al. Two cases of thrombosis in patients with antiphospholipid antibodies during treatment of immune thrombocytopenia with romiplostim, a thrombopoietin receptor agonist. Seminars in Arthritis and Rheumatism. 2016;**45**:10-12

[34] Mulliez SM, de Keyser F, Verbist C, et al. Lupus anticoagulant-hypoprothrombinemia syndrome: Report of two cases and review of the literature. Lupus. 2015;**24**:736-745

[35] Vandamme S, Sarah E, Elst K, et al. Lupus anticoagulant hypoprothrombinaemia syndrome: An instructive paediatric case. Journal of Paediatrics and Child Health. 2021;**57**:443-444

[36] Sarker T, Roy S, Hollon W, et al. Lupus anticoagulant acquired hypoprothrombinemia syndrome in childhood: Two distinct patterns and review of the literature. Haemophilia. 2015;**21**:754-760

[37] Pilania RK, Suri D, Jindal AK, et al. Lupus anticoagulant hypoprothrombinemia syndrome associated with systemic lupus erythematosus in children: Report of two cases and systematic review of the literature. Rheumatology International. 2018;**38**:1933-1940

[38] Sreedharanunni S, Ahluwalia J, Kumar N, et al. Lupus anticoagulant-hypoprothrombinemia syndrome: A rare cause of intracranial bleeding. Blood Coagulation & Fibrinolysis. 2017;**28**:416-418

[39] Chen X, Nedved D, Plapp FV, et al. Fatal pulmonary embolism and pulmonary hemorrhage in lupus anticoagulant hypoprothrombinemia syndrome: A case report and review of literature. Blood Coagulation & Fibrinolysis. 2018;**29**:708-713

[40] Eddou H, Zinebi A, Khalloufi A, et al. Thrombo-haemorrhagic disease related hypoprothrombinemia-lupus anticoagulant syndrome revealing a light chains multiple myeloma. Journal de Médecine Vasculaire. 2018;**43**:325-328

[41] Leko M, Yoshida M, Naito S, et al. Lupus anticoagulant-hypoprothrombinemia syndrome and similar diseases: Experiences at a single center in Japan. International Journal of Hematology. 2019;**110**:197-204

[42] Galland J, Mohamed S, Revuz S, et al. Lupus anticoagulant-hypoprothrombinemia syndrome and catastrophic antiphospholipid syndrome in a patient with antidomain I antibodies. Blood Coagulation & Fibrinolysis. 2016;**27**:580-582

[43] Kobayashi N, Ogawa Y, Yanagisawa K, et al. Acquired immune-mediated von Willebrand syndrome accompanied by antiphospholipid syndrome. Rinshō Ketsueki. 2017;**58**:613-618

[44] Gambichler T, Matip R. Erythromelalgia and livedo reticularis in a patient with essential Thrombocythemia, acquired von Willebrand disease, and elevated anti-phospholipid antibodies. Annals of Dermatology. 2012;**24**:214-217

[45] Hanley D, Arkel YS, Lynch J, et al. Acquired von Willebrand's syndrome in association with a lupus-like anticoagulant corrected by intravenous immunoglobulin. American Journal of Hematology. 1994;**46**:141-146

[46] Dicke C, Christina K, Schneppenheim S, et al. Acquired hemophilia A and von Willebrand syndrome in a patient with late-onset systemic lupus erythematosus. Experimental Hematology & Oncology. 2014;**3**:1-6

[47] Viallard JF, Pellegrin JL, Vergnes C, et al. Three cases of acquired von Willebrand disease associated with systemic lupus erythematosus. British Journal of Haematology. 1999;**105**:532-537

[48] Cao XY, Li MT, Zhang X, et al. Characteristics of acquired inhibitors to factor VIII and Von Willebrand factor secondary to systemic lupus erythematosus: Experiences from a Chinese tertiary medical center. Journal of Clinical Rheumatology. 2019;**12**:25-31

Chapter 3

Genetic Characterization of the Factor VIII Gene

Alexy Maza Villadiego and Samuel Sarmiento Doncel

Abstract

Hemophilia A is an X-linked bleeding disorder originating from mutations in the Factor VIII (FVIII) gene. This is a cause of muscle and joint hemorrhage that can lead to severe disability. From the references attributed to Jews in the second century A.D. to the last few decades, hemophilia has improved its control. Developments in the safety of obtaining FVIII products, their efficacy, and early prophylactic treatment strategies aimed at preventing bleeding and joint damage have made this possible. Although the appearance of neutralizing IgG inhibitors against FVIII in hemophiliacs is an outcome that makes treatment difficult, their relationship with genetic mutations that can serve as biomarkers to help improve medical decisions is currently being studied. The immune system tolerates our own antigens and attacks some that are foreign. After exposure to Factor VIII, immune antibodies can be generated that inhibit the activity of exogenous FVIII, predisposing to bleeding despite treatment. By administering high doses of factor, or using biological therapies, bypassing agents, or humanized bispecific monoclonal antibodies, the inhibitors could be eradicated. Inducing tolerance and making the body identify the therapeutic product without attacking it again allow the response to Factor VIII. It is important to establish the predictors of ITI success at the time of starting treatment. This chapter describes the importance of identifying different types of mutations in the Factor VIII gene that contribute to our knowledge in predicting the risk of developing inhibitors. This will allow the implementation of individual treatment strategies in patients hemophiliacs.

Keywords: characterization, Factor VIII, genetics, variants, inhibitors

1. Introduction

Hemophilia A (HA) is an X-linked recessive inherited bleeding disorder, with a prevalence of 1/5000 live male births, in which there are reduced, dysfunctional, or absent levels of Factor VIII (FVIII), which is essential in the coagulation cascade. HA in females is rare and results from inheritance of homozygous or compound heterozygous alleles or chromosomal abnormalities [1].

Previously the diagnosis of hemophilia was made through biochemical analysis and functional mixture studies to recognize quantitative and qualitative deficiencies of specific coagulation factors. With molecular analysis of genetic material (DNA), the aim is to identify mutations, genetic variants, and other individual differences in the hemophilic patient, see their association with risk factors for developing inhibitors or anaphylaxis in response to infused clotting factor concentrates, determine carrier status, establish prenatal diagnosis, and, with this knowledge, incorporate clinical care strategies [1].

Approximately 30% of patients with severe hemophilia A will develop anti-FVIII antibodies (alloantibodies). Inhibitors generally appear ≈within 20–50 days of exposure (DE) following the first application of replacement therapy, these inhibit the activity of exogenous FVIII from an immune response that has several origins and involves genetic (non-modifiable) and environmental (modifiable) factors. The most important genetic risk factor is the type of mutation of the Factor VIII gene. This gene is a multidomain protein consisting of a heavy chain (A1-a1-A2-a2-B domains) that is noncovalently linked to a light chain (A3-a3-C1-C2 domains). The mutation causes dysfunction of coagulation Factor VIII, making bleeding management and surgical procedures difficult, and increasing patient morbidity and mortality. Among the environmental risk factors, the type of FVIII product administered is important. Plasma-derived factors have lower immunogenicity than recombinant FVIII, and of the recombinant FVIII, the second-generation, full-length ones appear to be the most immunogenic in previously untreated patients (PUPs). Von Willebrand factor associated with plasma-derived products establishes a lower incidence of inhibitor development than recombinant Factor VIII. Another important factor is the intensity of treatment. Other environmental factors, such as age at the time of first treatment, have also been postulated [2].

2. Mechanisms of inhibitor development: Immune response

Different cell types play a role in the origin of the anti-FVIII immune response. The production of inhibitors, which are high-affinity IgG antibodies, requires the activation of CD4 T-cells, particularly follicular helper T-cells that are specific for FVIII. The activation of T-lymphocytes carries activation signals of antigen-presenting cells. For T-cell activation to be triggered, one or more peptides must have epitopes that are capable of binding to major histocompatibility complex (MHC) class II (e.g., HLA-DRB1) on T-cell presenting cells. Antigens. If this class II peptide complex is identified by a T-cell receptor, the relationship between the class II peptide and the T-cell receptor leads to the increase and secretion of cytokines that promote the production of anti-FVIII antibodies, that is, the class change. And the maturation of affinity. Therapeutic applications of FVIII expose the immune system of hemophiliacs to amino acid sequences lacking in their endogenous FVIII, which can lead to the development of inhibitors as these sequences are recognized by effector T-cells [2, 3].

It is important to register the spectrum of genetic changes and mutations of the entire population in international databases. This will enable comparative studies of genetic variation frequencies in different populations, allowing for the identification of founder effect mutations and mutagenic hotspots characteristic of specific groups. The development of NGS sequencing protocols will enhance the identification rate of pathogenic variants associated with clotting factor deficiencies, thereby increasing our understanding of genetic diversity within the normal population. Although genetic diagnosis of inherited bleeding disorders has been available for several decades, these molecular diagnostic tests are not available in all clinical hemostasis laboratories as a routine study and are used as a complementary diagnostic modality making it challenging for the clinician without this resource to understand the association between an identified variant and a disease phenotype [1].

3. Brief history

Much time has elapsed since the first written references to what may have been the first cases of hemophilia, descriptions attributed to the Jews of the second century AD, in which Rabbi Judah, the patriarch, exempts from circumcision the third son of a mother whose first two older sons died of hemorrhage after removal of the foreskin, over the years there are many other references to bleeding disorders consistent with features we know of fatal hemorrhage following minor surgeries. Otto observed that males suffered from the disease, and the disorder was transmitted from unaffected female relatives to a proportion of their children, those affected were known as "hemorrhagics" [4]. In 1886, Sir Frederick Treves first described hemophilia in women, possibly a marriage between first cousins [cited by Ref. 5]. König cited by Bulloch and Fildes, in 1890 described joint involvement as the most characteristic symptom of hemophilia, which until then had been confused with arthritis, rheumatic arthritis, other types of arthritis, and tuberculous. Bulloch and Fildes published in 1911, a critical review of about 1000 references and case reports establishing more than 200 genealogies, distinguishing cases of hemophilia by sex, symptoms, and heredity from numerous other records of unexplained hemorrhages and establishing their view that hemophilia could only be transmitted through the female route, doubting the diagnosis in those families where the disease was present in males, unfortunately until that time hemophilia was considered a fatal disease and at that time few males reached reproductive age [5, 6].

The disease became more widely recognized when Queen Victoria of England (1837–1901) was a carrier of hemophilia. Up to that time, the disease was not known among any of her ancestors, so it is assumed that a spontaneous mutation occurred. His son Leopold, the Duke of Albany, suffered numerous episodes of hemorrhages with mild traumas, which left him on the verge of death, he married Helen Mophilia at the age of 29 and died in 1884 at the age of 31 after falling and receiving a blow to the head, his daughter Alice born in 1883 became Princess of Teck [7].

Alice and Beatrix, sisters of Leopold and daughters of Queen Victoria, were carriers of hemophilia. Alice married Louis IV, Grand Duke of Hesse, and one of their sons, Frederick, died of hemorrhage at the age of three, and two of their daughters Irene and Alix, also had hemophiliac children. Irene married her cousin, Prince Henry of Prussia, and two of their three children were affected by the disease. Alix, better known as Alexandra, the consort of Tsar Nicholas II of Russia, had a son, Alexis, who suffered from the disease [7].

Beatrix daughter of Queen Victoria married Prince Henry of Battenberg and two of their three children were affected by the disease, and their daughter Victoria Eugenia, married Alfonso XIII, the former King of Spain [7].

Addis in 1910 added to the characteristic symptoms, sex incidence, and family history initially proposed by Bulloch and Fildes', the laboratory possible in which there was a prolonged clotting time and the addition of a "prothrombin" preparation made from the blood of a normal person corrected the prolonged clotting of the hemophilic patient [8].

Later Merskey published a paper (1950) in Oxford where he described mild degrees of hemophilia in which the clotting time was normal, but the post-traumatic bleeding was prolonged. It could then be stated that a male patient could be diagnosed with hemophilia whenever he portrays an abnormal tendency to bleed throughout his life and showed a reduction of Factor VIII [9].

The key to treatment was the development of blood transfusion. The earliest record of its use in a hemophilic patient was by Lane (1840) in which the direct transfusion of blood from a woman stopped bleeding that had persisted for 6 days in an 11-year-old boy after strabismus surgery. Macfarlane in 1938 considered that it possible to temporarily replace an essential missing component of human preparations of Factor VIII was developed in the 1950s [5].

It was a long time since the publication in 1901 of the Surgeon General's possible the United States, which included a section on the treatment of hemophilia with various therapies, until before the 1960s, when the treatment of hemorrhage consisted almost exclusively of the use of whole blood or fresh frozen plasma when available, bed rest and ice packs [10].

A notable advance in the treatment with blood products was described by Professor Judith Pool (1965) who observed that when frozen plasma was thawed slowly, most of the Factor VIII activity remained with the fibrinogen, and it took time to dissolve. This so-called "cryoprecipitate" when centrifuged could be refrozen and thus stored [11]. This was the first time the plasma had been frozen in a centrifuge.

Cryotherapy, a more practical treatment, could be used effectively in hospital centers to treat bleeding events and major emergency or elective surgeries in patients with severe hemophilia A (HA), but due to its storage in the freezer and the time it takes for reconstitution, it was far from being a possible therapeutic alternative for large-scale use [10].

In the 1970s, pharmaceutical companies (Immuno, Hyland, Kabi, and Cutter) produced plasma-derived concentrates of Factor VIII (FVIII) that could be stored in refrigerators, easily restored, and administered intravenously with syringes instead of droppers. That was needed to apply cryotherapy, which led to the introduction of home self-treatment and, later, periodic prophylaxis on a limited scale, replicating the pioneering experiences in Sweden [10].

4. The molecular basis of hemophilia A

Hemophilia A (HA) is an X-linked, recessive, inherited blood disorder caused by mutations in the gene that encodes coagulation Factor VIII (FVIII gene). The Factor VIII gene is approximately 186 kb in length and on the distal arm of the X chromosome (Xq28) has 26 exons and 2332 amino acids. It is composed of six domains in two chains, the heavy chain with domains A1, A2, and B and the light chain with domains A3, C1, and C2 [12].

Approximately 45% of patients with serious hemophilia A (FVIII <1 international unit (IU)/dL) have a homologous recombination event within intron 22 of Factor VIII. Their noncoding copy sequences are not part of structural genes, and they are oriented inversely (Inv22-1 and Inv22-2). Other pathogenic modifications of Factor VIII found in people with severe hemophilia A include large deletions, missense variants, and, less frequently, missense variants and splice site variants. In the distal arm of chromosome 22, Factor VIII is a major deletion in the distal arm of chromosome 22.

The exogenous application of FVIII continues to be the mainstay of treatment of hemophilia A patients with acute bleeding episodes and long-term bleeding prevention in most parts of the world. Recently, nonfactor replacement therapy (humanized bispecific monoclonal antibodies, emicizumab) was introduced. Replacement of endogenous FVIII may lead to the production of neutralizing (inhibitory) alloantibodies against FVIII in about 35% of hemophiliacs with severe disease. This is one of the most common complications represented by FVIII replacement therapy. This is one of the most common complications representing a challenge to HA treatment and leading to a high risk of bleeding increasing morbidity and mortality by compromising the hemostatic efficacy of treatment. Ultimately, inhibitors render FVIII replacement ineffective for both episodic and prophylactic treatment, necessitating alternative treatments [13, 14].

The FVIII gene was cloned, and its protein-coding regions were sequenced in 1984. The mutations initially identified as causing hemophilia A were reported very soon after cloning of the gene. These initial alterations were mainly large deletions or point mutations that damaged specific restriction enzyme sites. The arrival of techniques based on the polymerase chain reaction (PCR) made it possible to identify a good part of the remaining mutations that cause hemophilia A [15].

As of December 2022, more than 3500 different pathogenic variants causing severe hemophilia A had been reported in international databases: Factor VIII Variant Database (Factor VIII- db.eahad.org, Human Gene Mutation Database (www.hgmd.cf.ac.uk) and CHAMP (https://www.cdc.gov/ncbddd/hemophilia/champs.html). The most common genetic defects causing HA diseases include intron 22 inversion (inv22) with a frequency of 40–50% and intron 1 inversion (inv1) with a frequency of 2–5%. This disease has a high degree of mutational heterogeneity complicating the diagnosis because it cannot be based on screening for a limited number of common mutations except for inv22 and inv1. In the study of Pshenichnikova [12]. In a study evaluating molecular analysis of the Factor VIII gene in the Russian population with hemophilia A in 273 patients, pathogenic variants were identified in 267 of them (97.8%). 101 different pathogenic variants were identified and 35 of them had not been reported. The majority were patients with severe/moderate HA out of 217 cases (81.3%) [12].

Other studies in hemophilia patient populations in other countries have revealed similar results Furthermore, in this study by Sarmiento et al., although it had a very small number of hemophiliacs analyzed, it was observed that patients with a history of positive inhibitors (n = 4) had high-impact genetic variants (nonsense and Frameshift). The association between heavy chain versus light chain domains and risk of inhibitor development was 75% (n = 3) for variants located in the Factor VIII light chain (p = 0.075), suggesting that domains at this location are associated with an increased risk of inhibitor development [16].

5. Mutations responsible for hemophilia A

5.1 CpG dinucleotide mutations

In some regions of DNA, a cytosine nucleotide is followed by a guanine nucleotide separated by a phosphate group in the linear sequence of bases along its 5′ → 3′ direction. (CpG = is shorthand for 5'—C—phosphate—G—3′), Genomic regions where CpG sequences occur with high frequency are called CpG islands. G and C nucleotides are twice as prone to mutations as A and T nucleotides, and this has been determined from the comparison of pseudogenes and their functional counterparts. This means that a CpG dinucleotide, where the "p (phosphate bond)" is present, would have a mutational range that is at least 10 times higher than that of other sites.

More than 30% of all mutations detected in hemophilia occur at CpG sites within the FVIII gene, which contains 70 dinucleotides [15].

5.2 Missense mutations

A missense mutation is a point genetic alteration in which a single nucleotide variation modifies the DNA, resulting in a sequence of three nucleotides encoding a different amino acid. Various missense mutations can impair mRNA processing in addition to protein functions. Missense mutations are the second most common reason responsible for severe hemophilia A (HA). Some of the most frequent missense mutations include the Arg372His change, which damages a thrombin cleavage site critical for FVIII activation; the range of FVIII activity in these patients has been seen to be between 3% and 5%. The missense mutation Ser2119Tyr substitution causes a decrease in binding to von Willebrand factor, leading to mild to moderate hemophilia A [15, 17].

Missense mutations can be located throughout the FVIII gene and have been described to alter all sites from the initiation methionine (codon 219) to the final codon (2332). These mutations affect approximately 1 in 10 amino acid positions, although some codons, mainly those with a CpG dinucleotide, undergo several different mutations [15].

The Factor VIII missense mutation p.R2016W (c.6046c > t) (HGVS numbering; reference sequences NP_000123.1 and NM_000132.3 for protein and cDNA, respectively). Located in exon 19 is one of the most reported amino acid replacements that is believed to alter splicing and is a candidate to affect the configuration of the FVIII protein, damaging it at different levels, which is congruent with the variable degree of severity of HA. It was revealed that this mutation alters both the secretion and activity of FVIII. Furthermore, the substitution of the nucleotide (c.6046 C > T) linked with the mutation also reduces correct splicing at the mRNA level, which contributes to a further decrease in the already decreased level of FVIII expected based on secretion and activity altered. Null mutations (e.g., intron 22 inversion in hemophilia A, large genetic deletions, termination codons, etc.) decrease or abolish protein synthesis and/or release whereas mutations that alter amino acid composition (nonsense mutations) may particularly affect protein activity in addition to reducing biosynthesis [17, 18].

5.3 Nonsense mutations

A nonsense mutation occurs in DNA when a substitution in the sequence of an amino acid results in a premature termination codon (PTC) instead of a codon specifying an amino acid. The new existing termination codon leads to the elaboration of a reduced protein that is likely to be inefficient. It is predicted that PTCs will lead to nonsense-mediated degeneracy (NMD) of the message and its hasty intracellular destruction in many cases. NMD prevents abnormal protein clustering that could result in a dominant negative influence on a normal allele [15].

Nonsense mutations account for about 16% of the point mutations that lead to HA (http://www.factorviii- db.org). These patients frequently manifest serious HA and a high risk of producing FVIII inhibitors. HA predisposes patients to reiterative bleeding, especially in soft tissues and joints, its severity is inversely correlated with FVIII:C activity [19].

5.4 Small deletions and insertions

Small insertions and deletions (InDels) are arbitrarily delimited as those whose size is less than 200 bp. This variant has been associated with severe disease, although some also present moderate disease [20].

In the study by Werneck, small deletions and large insertions/deletions of Factor VIII were responsible for ITI failure in patients with severe hemophilia A and high-response inhibitors. This study included 168 patients with severe inherited hemophilia A and high-response inhibitors (≥ 5 Bethesda units/mL lifetime). The analysis found that intron 22 inversion was the most frequent genetic alteration (53.6%), followed by missense variant (16.1%), small insertion/deletion (11.3%), and large deletion (10.7%). The odds of ITI failure in relation to the intron 22 investment were 15.5 times higher (odds ratio [OR] 15.50; 95% confidence interval [95% CI] 4.59–71.30) and 4.25 times higher (95% CI, 1.53–12.3) in relation to those who presented large deletions and small deletions in the Factor VIII, respectively [21].

5.5 Large deletions and insertions

The large Factor VIII deletions correspond to 3–5% of the variations found in patients with serious hemophilia A. Severe HA is distinguished by a high percentage of genes in which all or part of them are mobilized from their normal location in the genome to another location within the genetic material compromising Factor VIII. Genomic rearrangements are the consequence of three primary classes of molecular mechanisms: (1) The overlapping in the ordered succession of nucleotides between two similar or identical DNA molecules (nonallelic homologous recombination), (2) The joining of two nonidentical broken ends of a chromosome (nonhomologous non-replicative DNA repair mechanisms), and (3) Replication-supported processes (RBM) of DNA. Molecular characterization of deletion breakpoints shows that the nonhomologous non-replicative DNA restoration mechanisms and the mechanisms supported by the duplication of the DNA molecule appear to be the essential processes responsible for the large Factor VIII deletions. In addition, a possible critical breakpoint of Factor VIII DNA involved in non-replicative rearrangements has been identified [20].

A deletion alters/modifies the DNA strand by deleting at least one nucleotide in a gene. Small deletions exclude one or a few nucleotides within a gene, in contrast/unlike larger deletions that can delete an entire gene or several contiguous genes. The deleted DNA can modify/transform the function of the damaged protein(s). Large deletions are arbitrarily delimited as being greater than 200 bp in size.

5.6 Splicing errors

Splicing deletes the interruption segments known as introns from the unedited RNA copy of a gene, leaving solely the regions of the genome that end with an mRNA molecule and contain the information to produce a protein (coding exons). There are more than 200,000 introns in the human genome and, if spliced together incorrectly, cells will create defective proteins. Several diseases are known to be due to mutations that change the normal splicing model. Half of the mutations that cause human diseases modify the efficiency and pattern of splicing.

There are many mutations that cause HA and represent a high risk of developing inhibitors. Numerous unique variants of the Factor VIII splice site are found. Patients with replacements at conserved nucleotide positions are considered high risk. These mutations are usually corrected and restore normal splicing less frequently, resulting in the appearance of alternative Factor VIII isoforms that have premature three-nucleotide sequence (codon) termination. Although splicing alterations are included within the types of risk variants, their impact at the level of protein transcript generation has only been fully characterized in limited cases [22].

6. Factor VIII gene inversions

6.1 Intron 22 inversion

Between 40% and 50% of people with severe hemophilia A (HA) have the disease due to the Inv22 mutation. Despite being linked to phenotypic cases of severe HA, the Inv22 mutation is not a significant risk factor for producing inhibitors [23].

Intron 22 of Factor VIII extends a 9.5 kb sequence (int22h-1) that has two extragenic copies (int22h- 2 and – 3) to a distance of about 500 kb to 600 kb from Factor VIII. These copies promote intrachromosomal recombination mainly during male gametogenesis. Inv22 can be type 1, when it recombines the int22h-1 and int22h-3 copies, or type 2, when the recombination occurs between the int22h-1 and int22h-2 copies [15, 24].

6.2 Intron 1 inversion

Has a length of about 1 kb and has a homologous gene situated 141 kb toward the ends of the chromosomes its reiterative sequences recognized as the end of the chromosomes prevent chromosome breakage or damage. Both inv. 22 and inv. 1 are susceptible to intrachromosomal homologous overcrossing causing inversion of the intermediate sequence leaving the FVIII gene split into two parts of contrary transcriptional sense. The clinical consequence of such inversions is a severe HA phenotype without efficient FVIII protein. The alteration is responsible for approximately 5% of cases of severe hemophilia A [15, 25].

7. Prevalence of different mutation types in hemophilia A

In a population of hemophilic patients with severe disease, mutation analysis should include the inversion of introns 1 and 22 and subsequently screening of the coding regions of the FVIII gene in those patients who do not have this inversion. Many studies have evaluated and employed strategies in hemophilia A patients looking for their different mutations, one of the most effective mutation screening techniques is denaturing high-performance liquid chromatography (dHPLC). It is used in mutational analysis of the FVIII gene and is classified as the "gold standard" method, identifying point mutations in 96.6% and DNA sequencing of the entire FVIII gene of hemophilic patients.

In a mutational study performed in a population of German patients with severe hemophilia A, looking at the relative frequency of different types of genetic alterations, a predominance of missense mutations and intron 22 inversions was evident while relatively rare mutations were intron 1 splice site mutations and large deletions. Advances in mutation analysis of the FVIII gene have made it possible to identify alterations in almost all cases of hemophilia [15].

8. Factor VIII mutation type and inhibitor development

In the early 1990s, eleven mutations were identified that were responsible for most cases of severe hemophilia A. After finding that antibodies against FVIII exigens can be detected in 30% of patients, the need arose to study the relationship of their appearance with the genetic variants that determine hemophilia. Of these, the study by Schwaab and colleagues provided the basis for further analysis of the type of mutation and the development of inhibitors [13, 14, 26].

Since then, many multicenter studies have been conducted which have focused on FVIII intron 22 inversion and large deletions especially, in the severe hemophilia A patient population, finding that there is a significant relationship between the type of FVIII mutation and the development of inhibitors for which they have been called severe molecular deletions, while only approximately 6% of those with nonsense mutations or small deletions did so [13, 14, 26].

Another analysis in 79 previously untreated hemophiliac patients (PUP) with severe and moderate HA, who were treated with the same product (Recombinate), in which genetic variants were analyzed concerning the presence of inhibitors showed a higher incidence of inhibitors in hemophiliacs with severe molecular defects vs. the incidence of small insertions, deletions and nonsense mutations [27].

In the meta-analysis carried out by Gouw et al., from 30 publications that included 5383 patients with severe hemophilia A in order to evaluate the hereditary factors for developing inhibitors according to the variants in the Factor VIII gene [28]. In this meta-analysis, we searched for articles that compared patients with intron 22 inversions with other mutations and the risk of developing inhibitors and found an increased risk in patients with large deletions and nonsense mutations (pooled OR, 3.6; 95% CI, 2.3–5.7 and OR, 1.4; 95% CI, 1.1–1.8, respectively), also comparing the risk of splice site mutations and intron 1 inversions being similar (OR, 0.9; 95% CI, 0.6–1.5 and OR, 1.0; 95% CI, 0.6–1.5), respectively and the risk of individuals with nonsense mutations and small deletions and insertions was lower (OR, 0.5; 95% CI, 0.4–0.6 and 0.3; 95% CI, 0.2–0.4, respectively) [28].

9. Genetic predisposition to inhibitors

There are several lines of evidence suggesting a genetic predisposition for inhibitors to develop. A positive family history of inhibitors has been associated with a three-fold increased risk of developing inhibitors. Furthermore, monozygotic twins, who are genetically similar, showed a 90% match in relaxation to inhibitor status, higher than that detected in non-twin siblings. Even when the total antibody response, that is, both neutralizing and non-neutralizing antibodies, is considered, the proportion of concordant familial antibodies appears to be higher than expected [29].

10. Ethnicity

African American individuals with severe HA and an intron 22 inversion mutation had a 2.3-fold increased risk of inhibitor development relative to Caucasians (odds ratio = 2.3 [1.1–5.0, P = 0.04]) [3].

But the cause of this has not been fully elucidated. Six distinct Factor VIII haplotypes have been recognized, designated H1 to H6. Two of these (H1 and H2) have been identified in all racial groups, but three (H3, H4, and H5) solely in the black population and H6 only in the Chinese population [30]. Considering that concentrated FVIII - both plasma-derived and recombinant - contains primarily H1 and H2, it has been proposed that a mismatch between the Factor VIII haplotype of the patients and the infused FVIII molecule would favor the risk of developing FVIII inhibitors [30, 31].

11. Future directions in hemophilia treatment: Innovations and challenges

Being the Hemophilia A genetic disorder that produces decreases in the levels of Factor VIII, hemophilia A (HA) and FIX, Hemophilia B (HB), at least three out of four patients with hemophilia correspond are HA, and at least half of them are severe [32] for which factor levels are below 1%, leading to a higher risk of spontaneous bleeding and difficulty in controlling it during surgical procedures and traumatic bleeding [33].

The golden standard for the management of hemophilia over the past 32 years has focused on the replacement of the deficient factor [34], focusing on patients with severe hemophilia or patients diagnosed with moderate (1–5% UI/dl) with bleeding phenotype [35, 36] showing a reduction in bleeding episodes, however, this therapeutic strategy has been faced with the development of inhibitors against the exogenous factor applied with an incidence of up to 30%, decreasing the effectiveness of the treatment.

Innovation in coagulation factors has mainly occurred in recent years in increasing the elimination time with extended half-life factors (EHLF) with which it has been possible to reduce the number of infusions and the effectiveness [33]. In 2018, a recombinant human monoclonal antibody that bridges FIXa and FXa to restore the function of deficient FVIIIa was approved in the USA, as an alternative to the frequent administration of deficient FVIII, administered subcutaneously on a weekly, biweekly, or even monthly basis, demonstrating that it significantly reduces bleeding episodes [37]. Despite these developments in technologies to treat patients with hemophilia, evidence also shows that there is still a risk of bleeding and therefore joint damage [38].

In low and lower middle income countries (LIC/LMICs) 70–80% of hemophilia people lack adequate treatment. In these the use of industrially fractionated plasma-derived coagulation factor concentrates (CFCs), alternative recombinant products and fibrinogen concentrates are the drugs of choice for preventing and treating patients with bleeding in inherited bleeding disorders. The availability of standard, extended half-life recombinant CFCs and their bifunctional monoclonal antibody mimetics, has reduced costs in some high-income countries (HIC) and successfully managed to obtain competitive costs for CFCs. Unfortunately, due to limited resources In low and lower middle income countries access to these products are insufficient [39].

The recent inclusion of cryoprecipitate, pathogen-reduced (Cryo-PR), in the World Health Organization (WHO) Model List of Essential Medicines for adults (EML) and for children (EMLc) emphasizes the importance of allocating sufficient resources for governmental regulation of Cryo-PR as a treatment for acute bleeding in various inherited bleeding disorders (IBDs) reasonably safe and potentially more affordable in hemophilia patients when access to CFCs is lacking, distinctly in countries with a high prevalence of infections such as HIV, hepatitis B, and hepatitis C [39].

Existing controversy regarding the use of native cryoprecipitate. In low and lower middle income countries where virus safety measures may not be present, the use of native cryoprecipitate carries significant risks and a high prevalence of transfusion transmissible infections. When available Cryo-PR can be cost-competitive with commercial concentrates of fibrinogen, as well as plasma-derived and recombinant CFC. The Council of Europe (CoE) Guide recognizes native cryoprecipitate alongside Cryo-PR and high-income countries with stringent virus safety measures like the United States native cryoprecipitate is considered second-line therapy. The WHO listed Cryo-PR as an essential medicine and native cryoprecipitate as an alternative product. Low and lower middle income countries should drive efforts to ensure its quality and safety pending access to Cryo-PR [39].

Hemophilia is a disease that only affects one gene (Monogenic) [40]. Studies are being carried out to evaluate the effect of other genes that interact with Factor VIII at different points of its expression, which could favor or worsen the possibility of reaching the hemostasis. As this disease is monogenic, it facilitates the development of gene therapy, and the Factor VIII gene transcript is small enough to fit into an adenovirus.

Gene therapy has been used since 2011 in patients with hemophilia B, achieving a constant increase in FIX levels even 8 years later, observing a dose-dependent expression of the genetic transgene [40, 41]. This therapy consists of the transfer of a recombinant adenovirus (AAV), whose DNA is replaced by a bioengineered gene cassette, with a tissue-specific promoter and regulatory elements [42].

After intravenous administration, transduction occurs, producing endocytosis and import into the nucleus where the genetic material is released, achieving to express the therapeutic gene, giving rise to the FVIII or FIX protein [42].

We do not yet fully understand the impact of neutralizing antibodies against AAV [43] and liver reactions due to genotoxicity [44]. The studies have focused on patients without liver disease and without inhibitors, the latter being those most likely to present bleeding.

The exclusion criteria in most gene therapy studies have been in the pediatric population since an increase in liver size and loss of transgene expression have been experienced [44, 45]. This is a challenge for gene therapy since hepatocytes are the physiological site of FIX synthesis, and sinusoidal endothelial cells are the main site of FVIII synthesis in the liver [41].

Other limitations, include the initial expression of Factor VIII, which is highly variable and unpredictable, the gradual decrease in expression after the first 6–12 months, and the impediment of treatment when there are preexisting anti-AAV antibodies from natural infections [46].

Some of the results of gene therapy in HA began to be seen with the study of Savita Rangarajan et al. [47], where nine patients were infused with a single dose of adenovirus serotype 5 (AAV5), in which the B domain of FVIIII was eliminated, with follow-up for 52 weeks, achieving levels of 3 IU/dl for patients who received low and intermediate doses showing that the treatment is dose-dependent since for those who received high doses they had levels of 5 IU/dl between week 2–9. Six participants achieved levels greater than 50 IU/dl at one year, at week 22 the patients with high doses did not present bleeding. An annual reduction of FVIII dose from 5286 IU/kg to 65 IU/kg was also seen.

The study by Pasi et al. [48] showed sustained but decreasing expression of FVIII, with mean expression decreasing by 43% during year 2 and 10% during year 3, however the annualized bleeding rate decreased by 96%, from 16.5 per year at baseline to 0.7 at the end of year 3.

We can conclude that the answer for optimal treatment of hemophilia could reside in gene therapy once the following is achieved:

Control of Factor VIII levels, not only to achieve hemostasis but also to avoid thromboembolic events [42]. Increased alanine aminotransferase (ALT) has been an adverse effect of gene therapy, leading to a reduction in therapeutic effect. Currently, increases in liver values can be controlled prophylactically with corticosteroids [49], may require immunosuppressive treatment [46]. However, the effects of these must be considered, as well as the development of innovative anti-Adenovirus drugs and finally financing, which, while it is true that in a 10-year horizon it may be in advantage over prophylaxis, based on the cost-effectiveness study by Machin et al. [49] where 8.33 QALYs were provided at a cost of $1 million vs. 6.62 QALYs at a cost of $1.7 million with factor replacement therapy, without adequate long-term funding, its implementation would be difficult.

The possibility of achieving Factor VIII expression in mice with hemophilia A with hematopoietic stem cells (HSC) and in immunodeficient patients with the use of human CD34+ HSCs transduced with a self-inactivating lentiviral vector CD68-ET3-LV encoding ET3 a new F8 transgene had been demonstrated. Srivastava et al., published a single-center phase 1 clinical study involving five severe hemophilia A patients without Factor VIII inhibitors. Before entering the study, all participants had reported an annualized bleeding rate of at least 20 events. They underwent gene therapy by transplantation of autologous HSCs transduced with the CD68-ET3-LV Vector completed at least 6 months of follow-up and evaluated the safety and feasibility of this technology [46].

The median follow-up after genetically modified hematopoietic stem cell transplantation (HSCT), in which CD34 + -enriched HSCs were transduced with the clinical-grade lentiviral vector CD68-ET3-LV, was 14 months (range, 9–27). Factor VIII inhibitors did not develop in any participants after drug infusion [46].

Evidence of endogenous Factor VIII expression was seen as early as day 18 after infusion of therapy. One month after therapy, a positive correlation was observed between the number of vector copies and the level of factor activity. The level of Factor VIII activity on day 60 was between 4.0 and 36.6 IU per deciliter. No spontaneous bleeding occurred in any participant during HSCT or after gene therapy. Two participants suffered a minor car accident on days 173 and 302 post-transplant with minor cuts that spontaneously stopped bleeding [46].

This new gene therapy approach by transplanting, after myeloablative conditioning, autologous HSCs transduced with a lentiviral vector has limitations, including the complex and elaborate process of HSC collection and manipulation to prepare the patient-specific drug. Early results from this clinical study reveal a new treatment option for hemophilia A that can be offered to all patients, possibly at an early age, and that results in sustained improved expression of therapeutic levels of Factor VIII. Longer follow-up is required, additional clinical trials with a larger number of participants will be able to clarify whether these expectations will be met [46].

Acknowledgements

Thanks to Arianna Sophia Maza Yepes for her collaboration, and motivation to push me to write this chapter to Prof. Dr. Cees Th. Smit Sibinga, for giving me the opportunity to write the chapter and believing in me, of course to the Lord Jesus, without him I could not achieve anything. I want to express my most sincere gratitude first of all to God for life, to my family for their motivation and to Integral Solutions SD SAS for providing a conducive environment for research.

Author details

Alexy Maza Villadiego[1,2,3*] and Samuel Sarmiento Doncel[1,4,5]

1 Integral Solutions SD SAS, Integral Solutions Research, Bogota, Colombia

2 Santander Hematology and Oncology Unit, Hematologist and Oncologist, Bucaramanga, Colombia

3 Bucaramanga Emergency Clinic, Coordinator Publication of Clinical Studies, Bucaramanga, Colombia

4 Life Sciences and Health Research Group, Graduates School, CES University, Medellin, Colombia

5 Catholic University of Valencia San Vicente Mártir (UCV), Sevilla, España

*Address all correspondence to: almazz02@yahoo.es

References

[1] Swystun LL, James PD. Genetic diagnosis in hemophilia and von Willebrand disease. Blood Reviews. 2017;**31**(1):47-56

[2] Garagiola I, Palla R, Peyvandi F. Risk factors for inhibitor development in severe hemophilia A. Thrombosis Research. 2018;**168**:20-27

[3] Gunasekera D, Ettinger RA, Nakaya Fletcher S, et al. Personalized approaches to therapies for hemophilia (PATH) study investigators. Factor VIII gene variants and inhibitor risk in African American hemophilia A patients. Blood. 2015;**126**(7):895-904

[4] Otto JC. An account of an hemorrhagic disposition existing in certain families. Clinical Orthopaedics and Related Research. 1996;**328**:4-6

[5] Ingram GI. The history of haemophilia. Journal of Clinical Pathology. 1976;**29**(6):469-479

[6] Bulloch W, Fildes P. Treasury of human inheritance, parts V and VI, section XIVa, Haemophilia. In: Also Published as Eugenics Laboratory Memoirs XII, Francis Galton Laboratory for National Eugenics, University of London (UCH). London: Dulau and Co. Ltd.; 1911

[7] Ojeda-Thies C, Rodriguez-Merchan EC. Historical and political implications of haemophilia in the Spanish royal family. Haemophilia. 2003;**9**(2):153-156

[8] Addis T. The pathogenesis of hereditary hæmophilia. The Journal of Pathology and Bacteriology. 1911;**15**(4):427-452

[9] Merskey C. The laboratory diagnosis of haemophilia. Journal of Clinical Pathology. 1950 Nov;**3**(4):301-320

[10] Mannucci PM. Hemophilia treatment innovation: 50 years of progress and more to come. Journal of Thrombosis and Haemostasis. 2023;**21**(3):403-412

[11] Pool JG, Shannon AE. Production of high-potency concentrates of antihemophilic globulin in a closed-bag system. The New England Journal of Medicine. 1965;**273**(27):1443-1447

[12] Pshenichnikova O, Salomashkina V, Poznyakova J, et al. Spectrum of causative mutations in patients with hemophilia A in Russia. Genes (Basel). 2023;**14**(2):260

[13] Peyvandi F, Kavakli K, El-Beshlawy A, et al. Management of haemophilia A with inhibitors: A regional cross-talk. Haemophilia. 2022;**28**(6):950-961

[14] Oomen I, Camelo RM, Rezende SM, et al. International genetic and clinical determinants of the outcome of immune tolerance induction (GO-ITI) study group. Determinants of successful immune tolerance induction in hemophilia A: Systematic review and meta-analysis. Res Pract. Thrombosis and Haemostasis. 2022;**7**(1):100020

[15] Goodeve AC, Peake IR. The molecular basis of hemophilia A: Genotype-phenotype relationships and inhibitor development. Seminars in Thrombosis and Hemostasis. 2003;**29**(1):23-30

[16] Sarmiento Doncel S, Peláez RG, Lapunzina P, et al. Comprehensive screening of genetic variants in the coding region of *F8* in severe hemophilia A reveals a relationship with disease severity in a Colombian cohort. Life (Basel). 2024;**14**(8):1041

[17] Donadon I, McVey JH, Garagiola I, et al. Clustered *F8* missense mutations cause hemophilia A by combined alteration of splicing and protein biosynthesis and activity. Haematologica. 2018;**103**(2):344-350

[18] Castaman G. Hemophilia A: Different phenotypes may be explained by multiple and variable effects of the causative mutation in the F8 gene. Haematologica. 2018;**103**(2):195-196

[19] Martorell L, Cortina V, Parra R, et al. Variable readthrough responsiveness of nonsense mutations in hemophilia A. Haematologica. 2020;**105**(2):508-518

[20] Jourdy Y, Chatron N, Fretigny M, et al. Comprehensive analysis of F8 large deletions: Characterization of full breakpoint junctions and description of a possible DNA breakage hotspot in intron 6. Journal of Thrombosis and Haemostasis. 2022;**20**(10):2293-2305

[21] Zuccherato LW, Souza RP, Camelo RM, et al. HEMFIL study and the Brazilian immune tolerance (BrazIT) study. Large deletions and small insertions and deletions in the factor VIII gene predict unfavorable immune tolerance induction outcome in people with severe hemophilia A and high-responding inhibitors. Thrombosis Research. 2024;**242**:109115

[22] Famà R, Borroni E, Zanolini D, et al. Identification and functional characterization of a novel splicing variant in the F8 coagulation gene causing severe hemophilia A. Journal of Thrombosis and Haemostasis. 2020;**18**(5):1050-1064

[23] Ashfaq J, Ahmed R, Tariq F, et al. Frequency of intron 22 inversion in severe hemophilia A patients. Cureus. 2022;**14**(8):e28247

[24] Vega Y, Faguaga M, Abelleyro M, et al. Inversión de los intrones 1 y 22 del F8 en pacientes con hemofilia A severa y portadoras del noreste de Uruguay. Archivos de Pediatría del Uruguay. 2020;**91**(2):84-89

[25] Schröder J, El-Maarri O, Schwaab R, et al. Factor VIII intron-1 inversion: Frequency and inhibitor prevalence. Journal of Thrombosis and Haemostasis. 2006;**4**(5):1141-1143

[26] Schwaab R, Brackmann HH, Meyer C, et al. Haemophilia A: Mutation type determines risk of inhibitor formation. Thrombosis and Haemostasis. 1995;**74**(6):1402-1406

[27] Goodeve AC, Williams I, Bray GL, et al. Relationship between factor VIII mutation type and inhibitor development in a cohort of previously untreated patients treated with recombinant factor VIII (Recombinate). Recombinate PUP study group. Thrombosis and Haemostasis. 2000;**83**(6):844-848

[28] Gouw SC, Van Den Berg HM, Oldenburg J, et al. Factor VIII gene mutation type and inhibitor development in patients with severe hemophilia A: Systematic review and meta-analysis. Blood. 2012;**119**(12):2922-2934

[29] Bardi E, Astermark J. Genetic risk factors for inhibitors in haemophilia A. European Journal of Haematology. 2015;**94**(Suppl 77):7-10

[30] Viel KR, Ameri A, Abshire TC, et al. Inhibitors of factor VIII in black patients with hemophilia. The New England Journal of Medicine. 2009;**360**(16):1618-1627

[31] Schwarz J, Astermark J, Menius ED, et al. Hemophilia inhibitor genetics study combined cohort. F8 haplotype and inhibitor risk: Results from the

hemophilia inhibitor genetics study (HIGS) combined cohort. Haemophilia. 2013;**19**(1):113-118

[32] Srivastava A, Brewer AK, Mauser-Bunschoten EP, et al. Treatment guidelines working group on behalf of the world federation of hemophilia. Guidelines for the management of hemophilia. Haemophilia. 2013;**19**(1):e1-e47

[33] Miesbach W, Schwäble J, Müller MM, Seifried E. Treatment options in hemophilia. Deutsches Ärzteblatt International. 2019;**116**(47):791-798

[34] Nilsson IM, Berntorp E, Löfqvist T, et al. Twenty-five years' experience of prophylactic treatment in severe haemophilia A and B. Journal of Internal Medicine. 1992;**232**(1):25-32

[35] Manco-Johnson MJ, Abshire TC, Shapiro AD, et al. Prophylaxis versus episodic treatment to prevent joint disease in boys with severe hemophilia. The New England Journal of Medicine. 2007;**357**(6):535-544

[36] Manco-Johnson MJ, Lundin B, Funk S, et al. Effect of late prophylaxis in hemophilia on joint status: A randomized trial. Journal of Thrombosis and Haemostasis. 2017;**15**(11):2115-2124

[37] Mahlangu J, Oldenburg J, Paz-Priel I, et al. Emicizumab prophylaxis in patients who have hemophilia A without inhibitors. The New England Journal of Medicine. 2018;**379**(9):811-822

[38] Mazepa MA, Monahan PE, Baker JR, et al. US hemophilia treatment center network. Men with severe hemophilia in the United States: Birth cohort analysis of a large national database. Blood. 2016;**127**(24):3073-3081

[39] Epstein JS, Maryuningsih Y, Faber JC, et al. Inclusion of cryoprecipitate, pathogen-reduced, in the WHO model lists of essential medicines for adults and children: A call for action. Blood Transfusion. 2024;**22**(6):481-483

[40] Miesbach W, Meijer K, Coppens M, et al. Gene therapy with adeno-associated virus vector 5-human factor IX in adults with hemophilia B. Blood. 2018;**131**(9):1022-1031

[41] Leebeek FWG, Miesbach W. Gene therapy for hemophilia: A review on clinical benefit, limitations, and remaining issues. Blood. 2021;**138**(11):923-931

[42] Miesbach W, Klamroth R, Oldenburg J, et al. Gene therapy for hemophilia-opportunities and risks. Deutsches Ärzteblatt International. 2022;**119**(51-52):887-894

[43] Stone D, Wang X, Abou-El-Enein M. Biomanufacturing in gene and cell therapy. Molecular Therapy - Methods & Clinical Development. 2024;**32**(2):101261

[44] Jagadisan B, Dhawan A. Hepatotoxicity in adeno-associated viral vector gene therapy. Current Hepatology Reports. 2023;**22**(4):276-290

[45] Ozelo MC, Mahlangu J, Pasi KJ, et al. GENEr8-1 trial group. Valoctocogene Roxaparvovec gene therapy for hemophilia A. The New England Journal of Medicine. 2022;**386**(11):1013-1025

[46] Srivastava A, Abraham A, Aboobacker F, et al. Lentiviral gene therapy with CD34+ hematopoietic cells for hemophilia A. The New England Journal of Medicine. 2025;**392**:450-457

[47] Rangarajan S, Walsh L, Lester W, et al. AAV5-factor VIII gene transfer in severe hemophilia A. The New

England Journal of Medicine. 2017;**377**(26):2519-2530

[48] Pasi KJ, Rangarajan S, Mitchell N, et al. Multiyear follow-up of AAV5-hFVIII-SQ gene therapy for hemophilia A. The New England Journal of Medicine. 2020;**382**(1):29-40

[49] Machin N, Ragni MV, Smith KJ. Gene therapy in hemophilia A: A cost-effectiveness analysis. Blood Advances. 2018;**2**(14):1792-1798

Chapter 4

Hemophilia B

Cem Selim

Abstract

The bleeding disorder known as hemophilia B (HB) is caused by a deficiency or abnormality in the blood clotting factor IX (FIX) gene, which is inherited in an X-linked manner. This disease results from one of more than 1000 classified pathogenic variations in the FIX gene F9, and genetic missense and frameshift changes predominate. HB predominantly affects males, while heterozygous females may present with excessive bleeding resulting from random or nonrandom inactivation of the X chromosome. In addition, homozygous, compound heterozygous, and hemizygous females have been reported. Evidence of somatic and germinal mosaicism has been identified in F9 variants. The occurrence of antibodies to FIX therapeutic products (inhibitors) is rare and is influenced by the specific type of causative variation. Genetic therapy is currently undergoing clinical trials and involves the use of products produced by recombinant DNA technology. Heterozygotes, putative heterozygotes, and all affected individuals should receive genetic counseling that includes up-to-date information.

Keywords: hemophilia B, coagulation disorder, bleeding, factor IX, gene therapy

1. Introduction

Hemophilia B (HB) is an uncommon genetic clotting disorder resulting from mutations in the F9 gene, which manifest as impairments in the quantity and/or quality of the circulating factor IX (FIX) protein.

Historical records of a hemorrhagic disorder similar to hemophilia can be traced back to the second century AD. As per the Babylonian Talmud, males should not undergo circumcision if two of their brothers had died due to significant bleeding during the operation. In the twelfth century, the Arab physician Albucasis documented a family where males succumbed to death by excessive bleeding following small injuries. In 1803, John Conrad Otto, a physician at New York Hospital from 1796 to 1817, provided the initial medical account of hemophilia. This description explicitly acknowledged the presence of a genetic link between sex and the likelihood of early mortality due to bleeding [1]. The term hemophilia was first used in a description of the disease authored by Hopff of the University of Zurich, Switzerland in 1828 [2]. In 1820, Nasse provided the initial genetic description, asserting that hemophilia was passed on from entirely genetically unaffected women to their sons [3]. Hemophilia is commonly defined as a royal sickness. Indeed, it has been demonstrated that Queen Victoria, who held the throne from 1837 until 1901, was a carrier of hemophilia B. Initially documented in 1952 by Biggs and his colleagues from Oxford, hemophilia B was given the moniker Christmas illness in honor of the first sufferer [4]. Contemporary therapy for hemophilia originated in the 1970s with the widespread availability of freeze-dried concentrates including FVIII and FIX. Inactivated clotting factor concentrates obtained from blood donations subsequently infected thousands of individuals with the blood-borne illnesses human immunodeficiency virus (HIV) and hepatitis viruses, without their knowledge [5]. While the initial documentation of a successful infusion of a recombinant FIX product that effectively prevented infection predates 1989, the commercial availability of recombinant FIX concentrate did not occur until 1998. Over the past 20 years, pharmacological research in this field has made substantial progress, leading to the creation of recombinant products that are entirely devoid of proteins originally produced by humans, both in the culture media and in the final formulation [6].

2. Etiology and pathogenesis

Hemophilia B affects around 1 in 25,000 to 30,000 live male newborns. Similarly to hemophilia A, hemophilia B is present in all ethnic groups and its occurrence does not rise in any specific geographical region. Factor IX is a monomeric glycoprotein composed of 415 amino acids and relies on vitamin K for its synthesis. Prior to its release into the bloodstream, the precursor protein undergoes significant posttranslational modification. Numerous intracellular processes take place during translation, such as the trimming and elimination of the signal peptide and propeptide sequence, γ-carboxylation of glutamic acid residues in the Gla domain, partial β-hydroxylation, N-linked glycosylation, O-linked glycosylation, sulfation, and phosphorylation. The posttranslational modifications (PTMs) of FIX exhibit a wide range of diversity and complexity, and the precise roles of the majority of these PTMs are still uncertain. A comprehensive study of the structure-function interactions of FIX subdomains is essential for gaining insights into the genetic condition of hemophilia B, which is caused by F9 mutations through several pathways. The concentration of factor IX in plasma ranges from 4 to 5 μg/mL, and its half-life is around 18 to 24 hours. It is typical for the plasma activity of factor IX to exhibit a threefold variation. Factor IX, being smaller than albumin, is spatially distributed in both extravascular and intravascular compartments [7, 8]. Its activation is mediated by either the factor VIIa-tissue factor complex or factor XIa, which together produce the active enzyme factor IXa. Upon activation, factor IXa stimulates factor X when factor VIIIa, phospholipids (activated platelets), and calcium are present. Factor VIIIa is an essential cofactor that enhances the activity of factor IXa. Hence, a shortage of factor IX or VIII leads to a corresponding absence of factor X activating activity on the surface of platelets. Cofactor Xa and factor Va catalyze the conversion of prothrombin to thrombin when active platelets and calcium are present (**Figure 1**). The lack or malfunction of factor IX molecules can lead to the development of hemophilia B. The degree of clinical manifestation of hemophilia B is approximately proportional to the functional activity of factor IX [8, 9].

3. Molecular biology and genetics

The factor IX gene is located on the long arm of the X chromosome (Xq27.1). It is much smaller than the factor VIII gene, approximately 33 kb long, and consists of

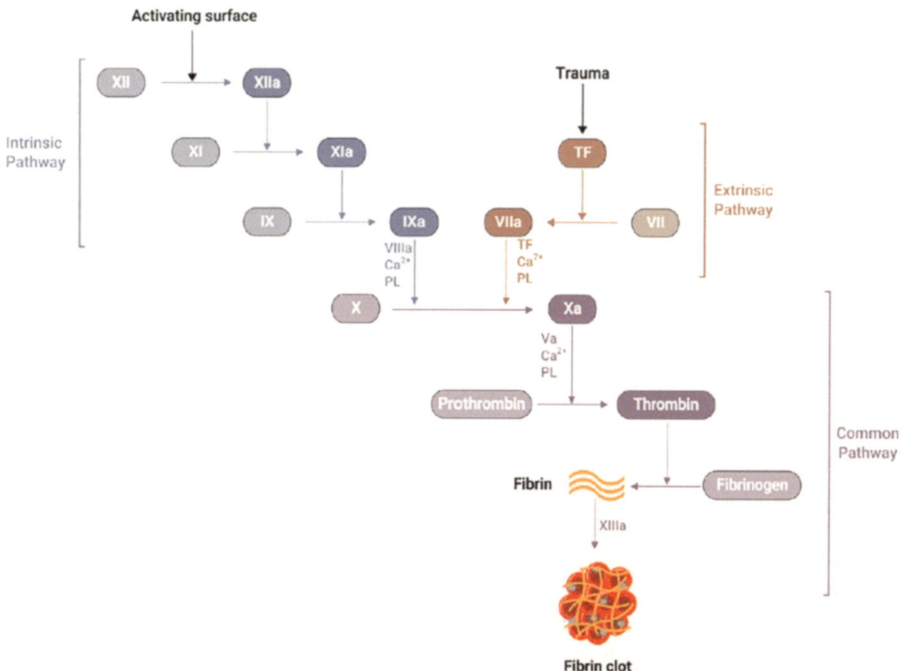

Figure 1.
Coagulation cascade [7].

eight exons and seven introns [10]. Eight exons transcribe into a 2.8 kb mRNA (NM_000133), which includes a 1.4 kb noncoding region at the 3′ end. The F9 mRNA's open reading frame (ORF) encodes a precursor protein of 461 amino acids (aa). This precursor consists of an N-terminal signal peptide (1–28 aa), an 18-residue propeptide (29–46 aa), and a 415-residue mature protein. The mature protein is subdivided into a Gla domain (47–92 aa), two epidermal growth factor (EGF)-like domains (93–171 aa), a linker sequence (172–191 aa), an activation peptide (AP, 192–226 aa), and a serine protease (SP) domain (227–461 aa). Exon 1 encodes the signal peptide for protein secretion from hepatocytes, exon 2 encodes the propeptide and the Gla domain, exon 3 completes the Gla domain and adds a hydrophobic helical stack, exons 4 and 5 encode the EGF-like domains, exon 6 encodes the AP, and exons 7 and 8 encode the catalytic SP domain [11]. The mature protein, belonging to the serine protease family, is synthesized in the liver as a single-chain vitamin K-dependent glycoprotein and is found in the blood as a zymogen at a concentration of 3–5 mg/L. The two main activators of this zymogen are activated factor XI (FXIa) and the tissue factor (TF)-FVIIa complex. The protein consists of a signal peptide that targets the protein for secretion from the hepatocyte into the circulation. The amino terminus of factor IX contains 12 γ carboxyglutamic acid residues that are necessary for calcium-dependent lipid binding. The activation peptide is cleaved from the zymogen form of factor IX by factor VIIa/tissue factor or factor XIa to yield the double-chain active enzyme factor IXaβ [12].

The factor IX database records more than 1000 distinct mutations or deletions in the factor IX gene, which include over 900 unique amino acid substitutions and a multitude of full gene deletions. F9 gene mutations manifest in both coding and noncoding sequences, encompassing promoters, introns, and 3′ untranslated regions

(UTR). A total of 1094 distinct mutations are distributed as follows: 897 (82%) occur in coding areas, 171 (15.6%) in noncoding regions, and 26 (2.4%) cover several regions. The database documentation includes 3218, 410, and 85 patients associated with these specific areas, respectively. Furthermore, the mutations in the coding area are virtually uniformly spread among the Gla, EGF1, EGF2, and SP domains, with a few instances occurring in the activation peptide [13].

The antigen-positive (cross-reacting material positive [CRM+]) variants of certain families of hemophilia B, similar to hemophilia A, can exhibit a range of clinical severity from moderate to severe. Although the antigenic levels of factor IX in these patients are within the normal range, their factor IX activity levels are markedly reduced. Over one-third (33%) of individuals with hemophilia B fall within this classification. Novel genetic variations have been discovered that affect several biological processes, including protein processing post-translation, gamma-carboxylation and lipid binding, epidermal growth factor (EGF) domain function, zymogen activation, substrate identification, and enzyme activity [14]. The F9 Cambridge and F9 Oxford homologs exhibit alterations in posttranslational processing that impede the cleavage of the 18-amino acid propeptide of factor IX. The F9 Chapel Hill domain demonstrates decreased activation of the zymogen due to disruption of one of the factor IX cleavage sites [15]. Within the F9 Vancouver variant, a point mutation causes a substitution of isoleucine with a threonine at amino acid position 397. This substitution disrupts the hydrogen bonding between threonine 397 and the carbonyl oxygen of tryptophan 385. This modification results in a decrease in the affinity of factor IX for factor X in a catalytic interaction that favors certain configurations. Proteins Hemophilia Bm is a defective protein that causes a prolonged prothrombin time (PT) only when the PT reagent is derived from the ox brain as the source of thromboplastin. Mutations in F9 that impact amino acid residues 180, 181, or 182 toward the amino terminus of the heavy chain, or residues 311, 364, 368, 390, 396, or 397 near the beta cleavage site of factor IX, can lead to the Bm phenotype [16]. The majority of affected persons have clinically severe illness.

Over 30% of factor IX mutations are in CpG dinucleotides. These genetic alterations frequently affect crucial Arginine residues, leading to a protein that is not functioning properly. Several mutations have been documented in several ancestral lineages, and some of these mutations originate from a common "founder." The genetic theory of X-linked recessive illnesses predicts that around one-third of the mutations leading to hemophilia B occur de novo. Novel mutations have been detected in the regulatory areas of the factor IX gene. Point mutations, characterized by the substitution of a single nucleotide with another nucleotide, are the predominant form of aberration observed in HB (**Figure 2**). They typically result from DNA polymerases erroneously incorporating an incorrect nucleotide during replication [17–19].

Genetic mutations in the F9 gene lead to the absence of FIX at several levels, including its gene structure, gene transcription, splicing, translation, posttranslational modifications, protein folding, and creation of functional complexes [13, 20]. Point mutations are present in around 88% of patients in the F9 variants database, whereas deletions, insertions, duplications, or indels are seen in slightly less than 12% of cases. Most deletions, insertions, duplications, and indels in the coding sequence cause a shift in the gene frame, resulting in the creation of a shortened or extended polypeptide with a changed sequence. A small proportion of these modifications lead to the inframe effect, which is defined by the removal or (and) addition of clusters of three

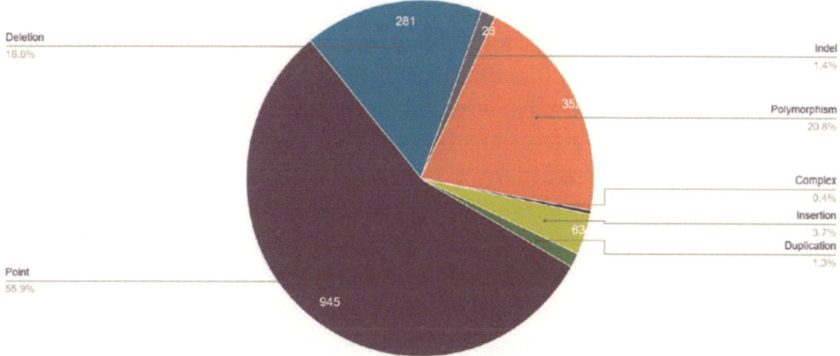

Figure 2.
Common mutations in hemophilia B. Available from: Factorix.com database.

nucleotides. The majority of patients with frameshift and inframe mutations suffer from severe hemophilia B disease. Most affected patients experience severe hemophilia B as a consequence of aberrant splicing caused by deletions, indels, and insertions in the introns 13. Roughly 2% of unique mutations affect multiple segments of the F9 gene and lead to total genetic deletions of the F9 gene, which ultimately cause severe hemophilia B. Moreover, it is crucial to note that individuals with significant deletions stand the highest risk (43%) of acquiring inhibitors [8]. Point mutations in hemophilia B patients represent a spectrum of bleeding phenotypes, varying in severity from moderate to severe. Multifactorial mechanisms contribute to the development of FIX insufficiency. Conventionally, point mutations in the promoter region cause hemophilia B Leyden8, but variations in the exons lead to missense, nonsense, or silent mutations. Point mutations occurring in introns induce aberrant splicing [20].

> Mutations in the 5′ promoter region lead to the hemophilia B Leyden phenotype. This disorder is characterized by very low levels of factor IX antigen and activity at birth and in early childhood. Factor IX levels gradually rise to 60% or more of normal after puberty, probably caused by an age-related stability element/age-related increase element-mediated genetic mechanism [21].

The mode of inheritance for hemophilia B is analogous to that of hemophilia A. All daughters of males who are affected are obligate carriers, while all male offspring are of normal genetic makeup. Among female carriers, the factor IX levels may vary between 10% and 100% of the normal range, with an average level of around 50%. Insufficient levels of factor IX activity, below 25% of the normal range, can lead to irregular bleeding, particularly following trauma and surgery [10].

4. Clinical

The clinical manifestations of hemophilia are associated with bleeding caused by compromised hemostasis, secondary effects of bleeding, or difficulties arising from the administration of coagulation factor. Infants afflicted with severe hemophilia commonly manifest signs during the initial 18 months of their lives, including facile bruising, bleeding in the joints, bleeding from mouth injuries, or bleeding after medical procedures. Typically, neonates with severe hemophilia do not have substantial bleeding even during delivery without the use of medical instruments. Hemophilia of mild severity can go unreported many times, particularly in the absence of a family history or if the family history is not disclosed, even if the family history is positive. Individuals diagnosed with hemophilia frequently have a documented familial predisposition and can encounter hemorrhaging in any anatomical region. The place of beginning bleeding is determined by the severity of the disease and the hemostatic difficulties experienced over the course of one's lifetime. Typical bleeding locations in neonates encompass the central nervous system, extracranial regions such as cephalohematoma, and sites of medical intervention such as circumcision, heel sticks, and venipunctures. Approximately 3 to 5 percent of newborns with severe hemophilia experience episodes of subgaleal or intracerebral hemorrhage during the perinatal period. Approximately 50% of individuals may experience severe bleeding after circumcision. As children undergo physical activity, the occurrence of bruises, joint bleeds, and other bleeding sites in the musculoskeletal system increases. Fractures to the frenulum and lips are frequently observed in young children, and forehead hematomas, sometimes known as "goose eggs," might serve as an early indication during the diagnostic process. Typical bleeding locations in older children and adults include joints, muscles, the central nervous system, and the oral or gastrointestinal tract.

Individuals diagnosed with severe hemophilia face an increased susceptibility to spontaneous and severe bleeding, with the initial occurrence that may take place as early as the moment of birth. Following trauma, they can encounter both acute and delayed bleeding, which can be either extensive or manifest as chronic seeping over a period of days or weeks. In contrast, extended bleeding from small skin lacerations is uncommon. As preventive medicine has become more widely used, the occurrence of bleeding episodes has reduced, enabling certain persons with serious illnesses to prevent significant bleeding events.

The clinical presentation of bleeding episodes in hemophilia B patients is indistinguishable from that in hemophilia A patients, and they experience fewer and less severe consequences compared to hemophilia A patients. Inadequate treatment of patients results in repeated hemarthrosis, which in turn may progress to chronic, debilitating hemarthropathy. There exists a direct correlation between the extent of FIX deficiency and the severity of bleeding outcomes (**Table 1**). Severe disease is sometimes described by factor IX levels below 1% of the normal range, moderate disease by factor IX levels between 1 and 5%, and mild disease by factor IX levels between 5 and 40%. Prevalence of factor IX inhibitory antibodies is far lower in

	Factor level	Bleeding pattern
Severe disease	‹1 IU/dL (‹%1)	Spontaneous joint or muscle bleeding
Moderate disease	1–5 IU/dL (%1–5)	Occasional spontaneous bleeding, prolonged bleeding after minor trauma or surgery
Mild disease	5–40 IU/dL (%5–40)	Spontaneous bleeding is not expected, severe bleeding may occur with major trauma or surgery.

Table 1.
Possible bleeding degrees according to factor level.

hemophilia B patients compared to hemophilia A patients and is extremely uncommon in cases of nonsevere disease. Merely 3% of those who are significantly affected develop inhibitors [22, 23].

5. Diagnosis

There exists a direct correlation between the age at which patients with hemophilia B are diagnosed and the degree of factor absence they experience. A diagnosis of severe hemophilia is often established when the child is less than 2 years old. In individuals with moderate hemophilia B, the diagnosis is typically established between the ages of 2 and 5. However, in cases of mild deficiency, the diagnosis is commonly made later in life, often for unintended reasons such as bleeding after trauma or surgery, or preoperative screening. A diagnosis of hemophilia B is established by clinical observations, family medical history, and suitable testing methods. Given that repeated bleeding episodes are very similar in different coagulopathies, it is essential to do proper laboratory testing to ensure precise and prompt identification of the disorders [24].

In hemophilia B, the complete blood count (CBC) is within normal range; nonetheless, a reduction in hemoglobin concentration may be observed when there is a high frequency and intensity of bleeding. In screening coagulation tests, the antiplatelet time (aPTT) is adjusted according to the extent of the reduction in factor VIII (FIX) activity, often assessed by a one-stage coagulation diagnostic. The prothrombin time is within the usual range. It is important to differentiate the diagnosis of hemophilia B from vitamin K insufficiency, heparin use, contamination in the sample tube, VWD, and hemophilia A, as these factors might lead to a prolongation of the apparent plasma transfer time (aPTT). The assessment of FIX activity level in hemophilia B should be conducted by factor testing. There are two techniques for evaluating FIX activity: the one-stage coagulation test using the antiplatelet assay (aPTT) and the chromogenic test. The first technique is conventionally a widely employed and much favored approach [25, 26].

To conduct the FIX clotting test (FIX:C), blood must be obtained in citrated tubes and promptly subjected to centrifugation at 2000 × g for 20 minutes. Next, the plasma is isolated and cryopreserved at −70°C. Post-thawing, the concentration of FIX:C can be quantified using either a one-stage or a chromogenic assay. The single-stage assay is a technique based on aPTT and is the most commonly used one. Plasma deficient in FIX and plasma from patients are pre-incubated with aPTT reagent for a duration of 3–50 minutes. Following the addition of calcium, it is necessary to monitor the clotting time. The plasma clotting time of the patient is compared to a standard curve derived from plasma samples with measured FIX activity. For the analysis of parallism between standard dilutions and patient plasma dilutions, it is necessary to measure a minimum of three dilutions of each patient's plasma. Parallel alignment of the two lines is expected unless an inhibitor is present. The chromogenic assay has two stages: firstly, a reaction mixture including FXIa, thrombin, phospholipid, and calcium chloride is introduced into the patient's plasma with an unspecified FIX activity. Quantification of produced FXa is directly related to the remaining plasma FIX. In the second stage, the peptide cleavage of a particular peptide of FXa, namely the nitroanilin sub-stratum, is quantitatively determined. The photometric analysis of generated p-nitroanilin is conducted at an absorbance length of 405 nm. According to a standard curve, the color produced is exactly proportional to the quantity of functional FIX present in the plasma [27, 28].

According to the research conducted by Kihlberg et al., there was no difference observed in the outcomes of the two activity test approaches among patients with severe factor deficit in hemophilia B. Conversely, in individuals with mild hemophilia B who had genetic abnormalities in the N-terminus of the activation peptide and propeptide domains of FIX, the levels of FIX were shown to be elevated in the chromogenic test as compared to the one-stage technique [27].

In cases when treatment fails to produce a desired effect or when there is suspicion of an inhibitor, a mixing test is conducted. Once the combination has been incubated at 37°C for 1 hour, the aPTT is conducted. If there is no aPTT correction in the combination, it suggests the existence of an inhibitor, and hence the Nijmegen test is required to establish the inhibitor titer. One inhibitor unit is the quantity of inhibitor required to deactivate 50% or 0.5 units of FIX activity for a duration of 10 minutes at a temperature of 37°C. This evaluation facilitates accurate decision-making for the treatment of patients with hemophilia B with inhibitors (**Figure 3**) [29, 30].

If the mother is confirmed to be a carrier of hemophilia B, it is possible to do chorionic villus sampling (CVS) and amniocentesis to screen the growing fetus. For such instances, it is advisable to do coagulation tests postnatally in order to ascertain the serum levels of clotting factors. Given that normal FIX levels are often achieved around 6 months following birth, interpreting FIX values at birth might be challenging. Thus, a little reduction in FIX levels at birth does not imply the presence of hemophilia B, but a substantial reduction in FIX levels (less than 1 U/dL) is indicative of the genetic condition. Through molecular analysis, the existence of the condition can be verified and significant information regarding carrier identification, prenatal

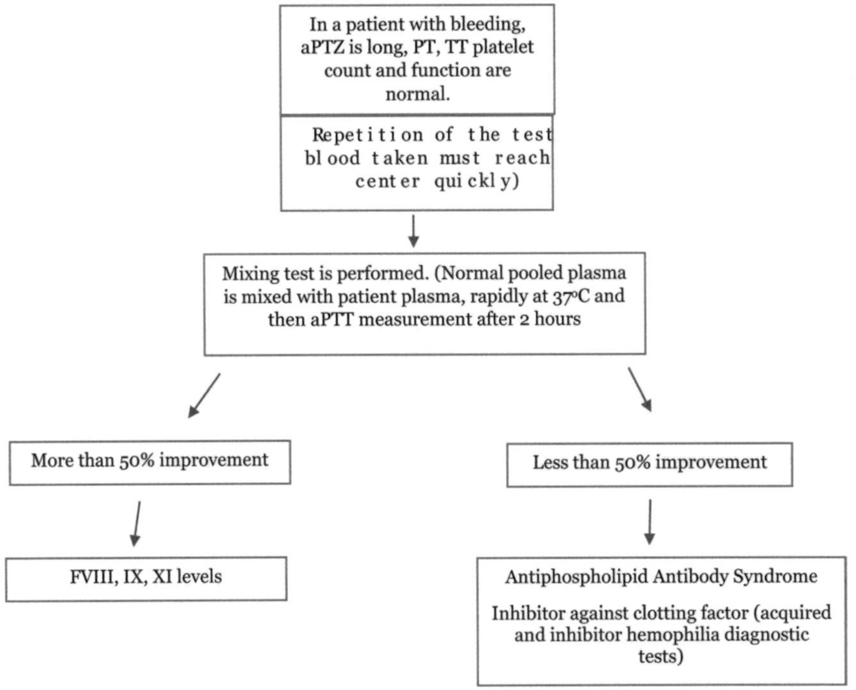

Figure 3.
Hemophilia B diagnostic algorithm (aPTT: Activated partial thromboplastin time, PT: Prothrombin time, TT: Thrombin time, FVIII: Factor VIII, FIX: Factor IX, FXI: Factor XI).

diagnosis (PND), and prediction of inhibitor development can be obtained, thus assisting in the treatment of the disorder [29]. Complete sequencing of the F9 gene is necessary for molecular diagnosis due to the absence of recognized common mutations in the gene. Polymerase chain reaction (PCR) DNA amplification followed by direct sequencing is a widely accepted standardized technique for molecular investigation. However, this technology is unable to identify significant deletions or other significant abnormalities caused by the existence of additional normal alleles. The detection of F9 gene mutations can be achieved *via* multiplex ligation-dependent probe amplification (MLPA) and multiplex amplifiable probe hybridization (MAPH) [31, 32].

6. Treatment

The cornerstone of hemophilia B therapy is factor IX substitution. There are several items available (**Table 2**). Traditional factor IX-containing preparations are commonly referred to as "prothrombin complex concentrates." Formulated from extensive collections of human plasma (from several thousand donors), these products include factor IX, prothrombin, factors VII and X, as well as proteins C and S. Furthermore, the products may include trace quantities of activated factors, namely factors VIIa, IXa, and Xa. A number of these items have been linked to thromboembolic events, likely due to contamination with the active components. Prior studies have documented instances of deep vein thrombosis (DVT) and disseminated intravascular coagulation in patients who have been administered high doses of prothrombin complex concentrates. However, it seems that these adverse effects are less common with the purified factor IX products now on the market compared to previous formulations. Prothrombin complex concentrates, while being more cost-effective than highly purified factor IX concentrates, are no longer the most suitable option for replacement therapy in hemophilia B. Excessive factor IX levels over 50% of the normal range should be avoided while using prothrombin complex concentrates for replacement therapy in order to reduce the risk of thrombosis. The use of these products in individuals with factor IX deficiency and compromised liver function may pose risks due to the inadequate clearance of activated factors contaminated by these preparations by a sick liver, which may lead to the induction of throstasis [22, 23].

Commercial product name	Storage conditions
Aimafix- Betafact- Reblenine 500 IU/10 mL	Must be stored between 2 and 8°C throughout shelf life.
Immunine- Berinin B 600 IU/5 mL 1200 IU/10 mL	It can be stored at room temperature (up to 25°C) for a period not exceeding 3 months without interruption, between 2 and 8°C throughout its shelf life.
Octanine F- Nonafact 500 IU/5 mL 1000 IU/10 mL	Must be stored between 2 and 8°C throughout shelf life.
Benefix (recombinant) 1000 IU/5 mL	It should be stored at room temperature between 2 and 8°C or below 30°C during its shelf life.

Table 2.
Some plasma-derived and recombinant FIX concentrates used.

Prophylaxis with plasma-derived FIX or recombinant standard half-life FIX (SHL rFIX) replacement products, such as nonacog alfa (BeneFIX®), nonacog gamma (Rixubis®), or trenonacog alfa (IXinity®), usually requires once or twice weekly injections. To alleviate this burden for patients, extended half-life (EHL) FIX products have been developed, including N9-GP (nonacog beta pegol; Rebinyn®/Refixia®), rIX-FP (albutrepenonacog alfa; Idelvion®), and rFIXFc (eftrenonacog alfa; Alprolix®). EHL products, compared to SHL products, offer enhanced bleed protection with once-weekly dosing and can sustain therapeutic trough levels of FIX with less frequent administration. Dose intervals of over 7 days with EHL products could enhance patient compliance and decrease factor consumption while preserving effectiveness [22, 23].

Dosage calculations for all factor IX products differ from those used in hemophilia A because intravascular recovery of factor IX is only about 50% and recovery with the recombinant product is even lower. The reason for this finding is not clear, but since factor IX binds to type IV collagen, a component of the vascular wall, adsorption of infused factor IX may contribute to decreased recovery. The factor IX dose can be estimated by assuming that 1 U of factor IX per kilogram of body weight increases circulating factor IX by 1% of normal or 0.01 U/mL. Therefore, to achieve 100% of normal in a severely affected patient (using only highly purified factor IX products), 100 U of factor IX per kilogram of body weight should be given as a bolus, followed by half this amount every 12 to 18 hours (**Table 3**). Dosing should be monitored by

Bleeding site	Hemophilia B	
	Desired level (IU/dL)	**Duration**
Hemarthrosis	40–60	1–2 days, longer if response is not sufficient
Intramuscular bleeding (except iliopsoas)	40–60	2–3 days, longer if response is not satisfactory
Iliopsoas bleeding *Beginning **Continue	*60–80 **30–60	*1–2 day/days **3–5 days (can be extended)
CNS/Head Trauma *Beginning **Continue	*60–80 **30	*1–7 days **8–21 days
Throat/Neck *Beginning **Continue	*60–80 **30	*1–7 day/days **8–14 days
Gastrointestinal system *Beginning **Continue	*60–80 **30	*1–6 day/days **7–14 days
Urinary system	40	3–5 days
Deep cut	40	5–7 days
Surgery (major) *Pre-procedure **Post-procedure	*60–80 **40–60 **30–50 **20–40	1–3 day/days 4–6 days 7–14 days

Table 3.
Bleeding site, treatment dose, and duration [22, 23, 33].

factor IX assays before and after bolus administration. Factor IX may also be administered as a continuous infusion after bolus administration in hospitalized patients. The standard half-life factor IX dose to be infused per hour can be estimated based on a factor IX half-life of 18 to 24 hours. Thus, in a 60-kg adult receiving highly purified factor IX, 6000 U of factor IX should raise the factor IX level to approximately 100% of normal. The level decreases by approximately 50% over the next 12 to 18 hours. Therefore, the patient requires approximately 3000 U of factor IX during this period, or 250 U of factor IX per hour by infusion. These calculations are only estimates of average responses, so factor IX dosing should be monitored by factor IX assays and the dose adjusted as appropriate.
Prophylactic treatment for hemophilia B may be attempted in selected individuals in the same manner as described for patients with hemophilia A. The prophylactic dose of factor IX with a standard half-life is 25 to 40 Units/kg body weight twice weekly or 50 to 100 Units/kg every 7 to 14 days if extended half-life products are used [22, 33, 34].

Tooth extraction, arthroscopy, lumbar puncture, endoscopy, bronchoscopy, synovectomy, bone marrow aspiration-biopsy, catheter insertion-removal, skin suturing-removal are minor procedures, while circumcision, organ system operations, and liver biopsy are major procedures.

6.1 Patient with inhibitor and treatment

One Bethesda unit (BU/mL) is the inhibitor titer that neutralizes 50 of 100% factor activity. An inhibitor titer of <5 BU/mL is called a low-titer inhibitor, and ≥ 5 BU/mL is called a high-titer inhibitor.

Hemophilia B individuals have an inhibitor development rate of 3%, and the two most significant etiologies found to yet are medication exposure and preexisting genetic alterations. Neutralization of the factor IX inhibitor is likely possible when the inhibitor titer is below 5 BU/mL, by the administration of substantial quantities of highly purified factor IX concentrates. It is recommended that individuals experiencing acute bleeding utilize the same medications used to bypass factor VIII inhibitors when the inhibitor titer is higher than 5 BU/mL. Administration of recombinant factor VIIa intravenously at intervals of 2 to 3 hours is recommended in doses ranging from 90 to 120 mcg per kilogram of body weight. As an alternative, doses of 50 to 100 U per kilogram of body weight every 8 to 12 hours (not to exceed 200 U/kg per day) can be administered of FEIBA, or inactive prothrombin complex concentrates. To induce immunological tolerance in patients with hemophilia B, daily infusions of pure factor IX preparations may be administered. Substantial side effects, including anaphylaxis and nephrotic syndrome, have been seen in seriously afflicted patients taking inhibitors. The nephrotic syndrome might be temporary and cured by stopping the supply of factor IX. The etiology of the nephrotic syndrome remains unknown. Anaphylaxis and hemorrhage in patients with hemophilia B and factor IX antibodies who receive factor IX infusions should be managed with a combination of inactivated prothrombin complex concentrates and factor VIIa concentrates, as FEIBA contains factor IX [22, 23, 35].

6.2 Current therapies

Successful transplantation of normal livers into people with hemophilia A or B has led to a complete cure for the hemophilic disorder. Nevertheless, due to the complexities associated with transplantation, it cannot be regarded as a legitimate therapeutic choice for the treatment of hemophilia in itself. A monogenetic disorder, hemophilia B is characterized by clinical symptoms resulting from the absence or malfunction of a single protein. Even modest elevations of factor IX levels can significantly improve the illness phenotype, making complete normalization unnecessary. Subcellular synthesis of factor IX is possible in cells other than the ones where it is typically generated (**Table 4**).

> Management of cardiovascular disease in the hemophilia population is challenging. The use of antiplatelet therapy appears safe in individuals with mild to moderate factor deficiency; however, for severely factor deficient patients, factor IX prophylaxis should be used. For anticoagulation with heparin or vitamin K antagonists, factor IX trough levels above 0.25 U/L are recommended. For the treatment of acute coronary syndromes and arrhythmias requiring intervention, factor IX should be administered at levels above 80–100%. Radial artery access is preferred to drug-eluting stents over femoral artery access and bare-metal stents. In patients requiring valve replacement, a biologic valve should be replaced instead of a mechanical valve whenever possible [22, 23, 35, 41].

Fitusiran, a small interfering RNA, diminishes hepatic antithrombin synthesis, thus enhancing thrombin generation and promoting hemostasis. Administered subcutaneously, fitusiran can be given weekly or monthly. In a phase 2 study involving patients with hemophilia A or B, with or without inhibitors, fitusiran (administered as 50 or 80 mg once monthly) decreased antithrombin levels by 80% and correlated with a median annual bleeding rate (ABR) of 1 in patients without inhibitors (n = 19). For the 14 patients with inhibitors, fitusiran lowered the median ABR from 38 (before fitusiran) to 0.88,89 without any thrombotic episodes noted. The phase 3 program for fitusiran was paused after a patient with hemophilia A, not having inhibitors, experienced a fatal cerebral vein thrombosis following three doses (31 to 46 U/kg) of FVIII. This led to a risk mitigation strategy that advises using lower doses of FVIII or bypassing agents for bleeds. Subsequent to another thrombotic event, the fitusiran dosage was adjusted to aim for an antithrombin level of 15–35%, and the studies are still in progress [42].

The use of viral vectors is currently the most common approach for hemophilia gene therapy. Recombinant adeno-associated virus (rAAV) has become the preferred vector. Adeno-associated virus (AAV), a member of the Parvoviridae family, is a naturally occurring, nonpathogenic, replication-deficient virus. Due to the endemic occurrence of AAV, preexisting neutralizing antibodies are common and have a prevalence of up to 50%. These antibodies often cross-react with multiple AAV serotypes. In addition, the development of neutralizing antibodies after AAV-mediated gene transfer precludes re-treatment with the same vector based on current technology. This is a significant drawback but is offset by the selective tropism that allows targeted transgene delivery and the ability to transfect both dividing and nondividing cells. AAV is also a non-integrating vector, thus minimizing the risk of insertional mutagenesis. rAAV vectors are produced by replacing the 4.7 kb wild-type AAV genome

Study name	Patients	Regimen	Objective	Outcome
US chart review [36]	Mild to severe hemophilia N = 64	rFIXFc OD or PPX	Understanding the clinical characteristics and outcomes from the real-world management of patients with hemophilia B treated with rFIXFc is essential.	Patients transitioning to rFIXFc PPX from PPX with another FIX product either lengthened or maintained their dosing intervals. Those receiving rFIXFc experienced a reduction in weekly factor consumption by approximately 50% compared to pre-rFIXFc PPX. Additionally, overall ABRs, AsBRs, and AjBRs decreased following the switch to rFIXFc PPX. Most patients saw improvements or stability in treatment compliance.
European Chart study [37]	Mild to severe hemophilia N = 30	rFIXFc PPX	Detailed analysis of actual clinical results and changes in factor consumption for patients with hemophilia B transitioning from SHL FIX (either OD or PPX) to rFIXFc PPX.	Transitioning to rFIXFc was linked to decreases in annualized bleeding rates (ABR), particularly for individuals previously on standard half-life factor IX once daily (SHL FIX OD), as well as reductions in injection frequency and factor consumption.
B-SURE [38]	Mild to severe hemophilia, PTPs N = 91	rFIXFc OD or PPX	Describe the real-world usage and effectiveness of rFIXFc in OD and PPX treatment of hemophilia B	rFIXFc was linked to decreased annualized bleeding rates, less frequent injections, and lower factor usage.
PREVENT [39]	Mild to severe hemophilia, PTPs N = 47	rFIXFc PPX	The practical application and efficacy of rFIXFc in the PPX therapy of hemophilia B will be described.	rFIXFc PPX has been shown to offer effective protection against bleeding with low ABRs and injection frequencies while keeping factor consumption within the anticipated range.
B-MORE [40]	Mild to severe hemophilia, PTPs N = 106	rFIXFc OD or PPX	Describe the real-world usage and effectiveness of rFIXFc in OD and PPX treatment of hemophilia B	Not Completed

Abbreviations: ABR, annualized bleed rate; AE, adverse event; AjBRs, annualized joint bleed rate; AsBR, annualized spontaneous bleed rate; OD, on demand; PK, pharmacokinetic; PPX, primary prophylaxis; PTPs, previously treated patients; PUPs, previously untreated patients; rFIXFc, recombinant factor IX Fc fusion protein.

Table 4.
Current's rFIXFc studies.

with the desired therapeutic transgene. While the 1.5 kb factor IX gene is within the capacity of an AAV vector, the larger 7 kb factor VIII gene needs to be modified by removing B-domain sequences, giving a 4.4 kb gene to fit into this vector system. Additional modification of the expression cassette to increase human hepatocyte tropism and increased potency through the use of stronger synthetic liver-specific promoters and codon-optimized factor IX cDNAs have also been important steps toward more successful gene therapy. For the hemophilia B gene, the use of factor IX Padua (FIX-R338L) as a transgene has the additional potential advantage of allowing a lower vector dose, as this naturally occurring variant has a mutation characterized by 8- to 12-fold greater factor IX efficacy [43, 44].

Etranacogene dezaparvovec, a successor to AMT-060, utilizes the same recombinant AAV5 capsid and codon-optimized gene-expression cassette, altered by a two-nucleotide modification in the wild-type human factor IX sequence. This change encodes the naturally occurring human factor IX Padua (R338L) variant. The factor IX Padua protein exhibits 6 to 8 times higher specific activity compared to the wild-type factor IX. The HOPE-B study demonstrated that etranacogene dezaparvovec outperformed routine factor IX prophylaxis in several aspects, including the annualized bleeding rate (both overall and factor IX–treated), factor IX activity, consumption of factor IX therapy, infusion rate, and the annualized rates of spontaneous and joint bleeding. The increase in factor IX activity was evident from the third-week posttreatment and sustained for 18 months, with no cases of factor IX transgene expression elimination due to hepatocyte-directed immunity [45].

In a study in which a rAAV8 vector containing a codon-optimized factor IX (scAAV2/8-LP1-hFIXco) was administered to 10 patients *via* peripheral IV infusion, dose-dependent but persistent factor IX levels ranging from 1–6% were seen in all subjects after 3.2 years, with a 90% reduction in bleeding episodes. Long-term follow-up (6.7 ± 1.0 years) showed stable factor IX expression without late toxicity in all patients. Similar results were reported with a baculovirus-derived AAV5 co-FIX administered to 10 patients, with a 4–7% reduction in spontaneous bleeding. These studies showed increased liver function tests but responded to treatment [46–49]. In addition to monitoring late toxicities, long-term follow-up studies will be needed to address questions about the durability of factor IX expression over time. Strategies will also be needed to address how preexisting AAV may affect immunity and potential loss of factor expression over time. Early studies of non-AAV-based gene therapy using gene editing techniques such as lentiviral vectors and zinc-finger nucleases have shown promising results. Although hemophilia gene therapy has been an active area of laboratory and clinical research for over 25 years, there are indications that major advances in this treatment are imminent based on progress made in the last few years.

Author details

Cem Selim
Faculty of Medicine, Adult Hematology Department, Selcuk University, Turkey

*Address all correspondence to: dr.cemselim@gmail.com

References

[1] Otto JC. ARTICLE I. The Medical Repository of Original Essays and Intelligence, Relative to Physic, Surgery, Chemistry, and Natural History 1803 (1800–1824). Vol. 6, No. (1). New York: T. and J. Swords; 1815. p. 1

[2] Hopff F. Ueber die Haemophilie oder die erbliche Anlage zu todtlichen Blutungen. Munich: Inaugural-Abhandlung; 1823

[3] Nasse CF. Von einer erblichen Neigung zu tödlichen Blutungen. Arch Med Erfahrungen. 1820;**1**:385-434

[4] Biggs R, Douglas AS, MacFarlane RG, et al. Christmas disease: A condition previously mistaken for haemophilia. BMJ. 1952;**2**(4799):1378-1382

[5] Mannucci PM. Hemophilia: Treatment options in the twenty-first century. Journal of Thrombosis and Haemostasis. 2003;**1**(7):1349-1355

[6] Monahan PE, Di Paola J. Recombinant factor IX for clinical and research use. Seminars in Thrombosis and Hemostasis. 2010;**36**(5):498-409

[7] Mruthunjaya AK, Torriero AA. Electrochemical monitoring in anticoagulation therapy. Molecules. 2024;**29**(7):1453-1456

[8] Goodeve AC, Peake IR. The molecular basis of hemophilia A: Genotype-phenotype relationships and inhibitor development. Seminars in Thrombosis and Hemostasis. 2003;**29**(01):23-30

[9] Zimmerman B, Leonard AV. Hemophilia: In review. Pediatrics in Review. 2013;**34**(7):289-295

[10] Miller CH. The clinical genetics of hemophilia B (factor IX deficiency). The Application of Clinical Genetics. 2021; **14**:445-454

[11] Shen G, Gao M, Cao Q. The molecular basis of FIX deficiency in hemophilia B. International Journal of Molecular Sciences. 2022;**23**(5):2762

[12] Kurachi K, Davie EW. Isolation and characterization of a cDNA coding for human factor IX. Proceedings of the National Academy of Sciences. 1982; **79**(21):6461-6464

[13] Rallapalli PM, Kemball-Cook G, Tuddenham EG. An interactive mutation database for human coagulation factor IX provides novel insights into the phenotypes and genetics of hemophilia B. Journal of Thrombosis and Haemostasis. 2013;**11**(7):1329-1340

[14] Diuguid DL, Rabiet MJ, Furie BC, et al. Molecular basis of hemophilia B: A defective enzyme due to an unprocessed propeptide is caused by a point mutation in the factor IX precursor. Proceedings of the National Academy of Sciences. 1986;**83**(16):5803-5807

[15] Noyes CM, Griffith MJ, Roberts HR, et al. Identification of the molecular defect in factor IX Chapel Hill: Substitution of histidine for arginine at position 145. Proceedings of the National Academy of Sciences. 1983;**80**(14): 4200-4202

[16] Hamaguchi N, Roberts H, Stafford DW, et al. Mutations in the catalytic domain of factor IX that are related to the subclass hemophilia Bm. Biochemistry. 1993;**32**(25):6324-6329

[17] Bertina RM, van der Linden IK, Mannucci PM, et al. Mutations in hemophilia Bm occur at the Arg180-Val activation site or in the catalytic domain of factor IX. The Journal of Biological Chemistry. 1990;**265**(19):10876-10883

[18] Goodeve AC. Hemophilia B: Molecular pathogenesis and mutation analysis. Journal of Thrombosis and Haemostasis. 2015;**13**(7):1184-1195

[19] Goodeve AC. Laboratory methods for the genetic diagnosis of bleeding disorders. Clinical and Laboratory Haematology. 1998;**20**(1):3-19

[20] Melendez-Aranda L, Jaloma-Cruz AR, Pastor N, et al. In silico analysis of missense mutations in exons 1-5 of the F9 gene that cause hemophilia B. BMC Bioinformatics. 2019;**20**:1-13

[21] Kurachi S, Huo JS, Ameri A, et al. An age-related homeostasis mechanism is essential for spontaneous amelioration of hemophilia B Leyden. Proceedings of the National Academy of Sciences. 2009; **106**(19):7921-7926

[22] Srivastava A, Santagostino E, Dougall A, et al. WFH guidelines for the management of hemophilia, 3rd edition. Haemophilia. 2020;**26**:1-158

[23] Kavaklı K, Demir AM, Küpesiz A, et al. Türk Hematoloji Derneği. Ulusal Hemofili Tanı ve Tedavi Kılavuzu. 2021; **3**:34-89

[24] Dorgalaleh A, Dadashizadeh G, Bamedi T. Hemophilia in Iran. Hematology. 2016;**21**(5):300-310

[25] Kitchen S, McCraw A, Echenagucia M. Diagnosis of Haemophilia and Other Bleeding Disorders: A Laboratory Manual. Montreal: World Federation of Hemophilia Montreal; 2000

[26] Kizilocak H, Young G. Diagnosis and treatment of hemophilia. Clinical Advances in Hematology & Oncology. 2019;**17**(6):344-351

[27] Kihlberg K, Strandberg K, Rosén S, Ljung R, Astermark J. Discrepancies between the one-stage clotting assay and the chromogenic assay in haemophilia B. Haemophilia. 2017;**23**(4):620-627

[28] Kitchen S, Signer-Romero K, Key N. Current laboratory practices in the diagnosis and management of haemophilia: A global assessment. Haemophilia. 2015;**21**(4):550-557

[29] Mahlangu JN. Updates in clinical trial data of extended half-life recombinant factor IX products for the treatment of haemophilia B. Therapeutic Advances in Hematology. 2018;**9**(11):335-339

[30] Feng D, Stafford KA, Broze GJ, et al. Evidence of clinically significant extravascular stores of factor IX. Journal of Thrombosis and Haemostasis. 2013; **11**(12):2176-2178

[31] Sellner LN, Taylor GR. MLPA and MAPH: New techniques for detection of gene deletions. Human Mutation. 2004; **23**(5):413-419

[32] Kwon MJ, Yoo KY, Kim HJ, Kim SH. Identification of mutations in the F9 gene including exon deletion by multiplex ligation-dependent probe amplification in 33 unrelated Korean patients with haemophilia B. Haemophilia. 2008;**14**(5):1069-1075

[33] Santoro C, Quintavalle G, Castaman G, et al. Inhibitors in hemophilia B. Seminars in Thrombosis and Hemostasis. 2018;**44**(6):578-579

[34] Marchesini E, Morfini M, Valentino L. Recent advances in the treatment of hemophilia: A review. Biological Theory. 2021;**15**:221-235

[35] Wilde J, Teixeira P, Bramhall SR, et al. Liver transplantation in haemophilia. British Journal of Haematology. 2002;**117**(4):952-956

[36] Shapiro A, Chaudhury A, Wang M, et al. Real-world data demonstrate

improved bleed control and extended dosing intervals for patients with haemophilia B after switching to recombinant factor IX fc fusion protein (rFIXFc) for up to 5 years. Haemophilia. 2020;**26**(6):975-983

[37] Funding E, Lowe G, Poulsen LH, et al. Real-world effectiveness of rFIXFc prophylaxis in patients with haemophilia B switched from standard half-life therapy in three European countries. Advances in Therapy. 2023;**40**(9): 3770-3783

[38] Chambost H, Repesse Y, Genre Volot F, et al. Final data from B-SURE, a French multicentre study in patients with haemophilia B, evaluating real-world usage and effectiveness of recombinant factor IX fc (rFIXFc). Haemophilia. 2023;**29**(1): 57-58

[39] Bidlingmaier C, Heller H, Langer F, et al. Final data from the PREVENT study evaluating real-world usage and effectiveness of a recombinant factor VIII fc and recombinant factor IX fc in haemophilia a or B in Germany. Haemophilia. 2023;**29**:48-49

[40] Glosli H, Ranta S, Allsup D, et al. Interim analysis from B-MORE, a 24-month prospective, multicentre, non-interventional study on effectiveness and usage of recombinant factor IX fc (rFIXFc) in haemophilia B [ISTH abstract PB1153]. Presented at: ISTH congress 2022. Research and Practice in Thrombosis and Haemostasis. 2022;**6**(S1):e12788

[41] Calcedo R, Vandenberghe LH, Gao G, et al. Worldwide epidemiology of neutralizing antibodies to adeno-associated viruses. The Journal of Infectious Diseases. 2009;**199**(3): 381-390

[42] Whelan SF, Hofbauer CJ, Horling FM, et al. Distinct characteristics of antibody responses against factor VIII in healthy individuals and in different cohorts of hemophilia A patients. Blood. 2013;**121**(6):1039-1048

[43] Perrin GQ, Herzog RW, Markusic DM. Update on clinical gene therapy for hemophilia. Blood. 2019; **133**(5):407-412

[44] Nathwani AC, Reiss UM, Tuddenham EG, et al. Adeno-associated mediated gene transfer for hemophilia B. 8 year follow up and impact of removing "empty viral particles" on safety and efficacy of gene transfer. Blood. 2018; **132**:491

[45] Pipe SW, Leebeek FW, Recht M, et al. Gene therapy with etranacogene dezaparvovec for hemophilia B. The New England Journal of Medicine. 2023; **388**(8):706-718

[46] Miesbach W, Meijer K, Coppens M, et al. Gene therapy with adeno-associated virus vector 5-human factor IX in adults with hemophilia B. Blood. 2018;**131**(9):1022-1031

[47] Leebeek F, Meijer K, Coppens M, et al. Reduction in annualized bleeding and factor IX consumption up to 2.5 years in adults with severe or moderate-severe hemophilia B treated with AMT-060 AAV5-hFIX gene therapy. Blood. 2018;**132**(92):3476

[48] Schutgens REG, Voskuil M, Mauser-Bunschoten EP. Management of cardiovascular disease in aging persons with haemophilia. Hämostaseologie. 2017;**37**(3):196-199

[49] Tuinenburg A, Damen SA, Ypma PF, et al. Cardiac catheterization and intervention in haemophilia patients: Prospective evaluation of the 2009 institutional guideline. Haemophilia. 2013;**19**(3):370-377

Chapter 5

Perspective Chapter: Cerebral Venous Thrombosis – New Trends in Therapy?

Małgorzata Wiszniewska

Abstract

Cerebral venous thrombosis (CVT) is a rare disease of the nervous system caused by thrombosis of cerebral veins and/or dural venous sinuses, most commonly the superior sagittal sinus. In developed countries, the prevalence of the disease is estimated at 1.32/100,000 per year. It accounts for 0.5–1% of all strokes. CVT predominantly affects young people, with less than 10% being over the age of 65. Women predominate among young people, which is attributed to gender-specific risk factors for CVT. The increased incidence observed in recent years is likely due to greater awareness of the disease and the availability of advanced neuroimaging techniques, which enable accurate diagnosis even in atypical cases. The variety of symptoms, heterogeneous clinical course, and multiple causes of the disease make CVT a significant diagnostic and therapeutic challenge. Delayed diagnosis can result in life-threatening progression of the disease.

Keywords: cerebral venous thrombosis (CVT), anticoagulation therapy, MRI scan, computed tomography (CT) scan, hemicraniectomy

1. Introduction

Cerebral venous thrombosis (CVT) is a rare disease of the nervous system caused by thrombosis of cerebral veins and/or dural venous sinuses, most commonly the superior sagittal sinus [1]. In developed countries, the prevalence of the disease is estimated at 1.32/100000 per year [2]. It accounts for 0.5–1% of all strokes [3]. CVT predominantly affects young people, with less than 10% being over the age of 65 [4]. Women predominate among young people, which is attributed to gender-specific risk factors for CVT [5].

The increased incidence observed in recent years is likely due to greater awareness of the disease and the availability of advanced neuroimaging techniques, which enable accurate diagnosis even in atypical cases. The variety of symptoms, heterogeneous clinical course, and multiple causes of the disease make CVT a significant diagnostic and therapeutic challenge. Delayed diagnosis can result in life-threatening progression of the disease [5].

1.1 Risk factors

Important risk factors include congenital and acquired thrombophilia, inflammatory diseases, and cancer, which are also common to other venous thromboembolic diseases [5, 6]. The most common thrombophilias identified in patients with CVT were found to be the prothrombin gene G20210A polymorphism (in 6–20% cases of CVT), the FV-Leiden G1691A mutation (10–24%), antiphospholipid syndrome (6–8%) and, less frequently, protein C and S deficiency and antithrombin III deficiency (0–9%) [7]. A link between hyperhomocysteinemia and an increased risk of developing CVT has also been confirmed (OR, 4.07, 95% CI 2.54–6.52) [8].

Risk factors for CVT in women include hormone replacement therapy, estrogen oral contraceptives, pregnancy, and the postpartum period. The risk of thrombosis in women using oral contraceptives is up to six times higher and is further elevated in women with obesity [9].

Other factors that increase the risk of CVT include head trauma, arteriovenous malformations, neurosurgery, and infections in the head and neck, as well as obesity and chronic use of corticosteroids [9–12]. In some patients, more than one risk factor is identified, and in about 10–15% of patients, the etiology of the disease cannot be determined [4, 13]. It is worth noting that, although rare, CVT with concomitant thrombocytopenia may occur a few days to a few weeks after administration of the adenovirus-based SARS-CoV-2 vaccine. In such cases, consultation with a hematologist is essential, and treatment should be carried out in collaboration with them [4, 10].

1.2 Clinical picture

Disease symptoms can develop in an acute (<48 h, 30%), subacute (<1 month, 52%), or chronic (>1 m-c, 18%) manner [11, 14, 15]. The clinical picture is variable and depends on the location of the thrombosis, resulting from increased intracranial pressure and brain damage (edema, hemorrhage, ischemia) [5].

Signs that suggest a venous etiology of stroke include headache (in 90% of patients), optic disc swelling (present in about 28% of patients), co-occurrence of epileptic seizures (40%), disturbance of consciousness, a fluctuating disease course, and slow progression of symptoms, as well as bilateral involvement of brain structures [14].

In CVT, four main groups of symptoms are distinguished: (a) isolated intracranial hypertension (headache, reduced visual acuity, swelling of the CN II discs); (b) focal symptoms (paresis, epileptic seizures); (c) encephalopathy, with predominant disturbances of consciousness; and (d) cavernous sinus syndrome [5, 15, 16].

2. Diagnosis

The non-specific nature of the disease's symptoms causes diagnostic difficulties, often leading to delays in diagnosis. On average, the time from the onset of symptoms to diagnosis is 7 days [5, 11, 17].

2.1 Laboratory tests

While laboratory test results do not confirm or exclude thrombosis, routine blood tests—assessing morphology, biochemistry, and coagulation—are recommended when CVT is suspected, as they can help diagnose co-morbidities [5, 10, 18].

2.2 D-dimers in the diagnosis of CVT

In patients with suspected CVT, it is suggested to measure serum D-dimers, excluding patients with isolated headaches and those with a long duration of symptoms (>7 days). A systematic review of 14 studies evaluating the value of D-dimer determination in the diagnosis of CVT in 1134 patients confirmed its high sensitivity (93.9%; 95% CI 87.5–97.1) and specificity (89.7%; 95% CI 86.5–92.2) [5, 18, 19]. False-negative results were obtained in patients with isolated headaches in the course of CVT, long duration of symptoms (more than 7 days), and limited sinus involvement. There is a relationship between the extent of thrombosis and D-dimer concentration. D-dimer concentration decreases as the disease progresses. Therefore, as long as there is a high clinical suspicion of CVT, a normal D-dimer result should not be the basis for ruling out the disease [5, 13, 18]. Also, a mere elevation of D-dimer without any clinical symptoms is not sufficient for the diagnosis of CVT [5, 18, 19].

Diagnosis for thrombophilia (determination of anticardiolipin antibodies, lupus anticoagulant, protein C and S, antithrombin III, FV-Leiden mutation, prothrombin G20210A mutation) and assessment of homocysteine levels should be performed in patients in whom CVT risk factors have not been identified, with recurrent thrombosis, who have a family history of thrombosis, and in young patients [5–8, 19].

Examination of the cerebrospinal fluid (CSF) allows to rule out meningitis, which can also cause CVT, but in the absence of suspected inflammation, it is not helpful in the diagnosis of CVT. Slight pleocytosis and elevated protein concentrations may be present in the CSF (in 50 and 35% of cases, respectively). Elevated opening pressure is found in 80% of cases [5, 18].

2.3 Neuroimaging studies

The aim of diagnostic neuroimaging is to visualize an obstructed sinus/vein. It can also reveal non-specific lesions such as infarction, hemorrhage, or edema. There are three main methods used in the diagnosis of cerebral thrombosis: magnetic resonance (MR) with venography, computed tomography (CT) with venography, and traditional angiography [20–22].

CT scanning is commonly used as initial neuroimaging in suspected stroke, although it is a low-sensitivity method, and it is not always sufficient in the diagnosis of CVT. On this basis, thrombosis can be suspected in 30% of patients. An obstructed sinus or vein can be seen as an area of increased signal intensity (hyperdense), which in cases of posterior superior sagittal sinus thrombosis results in the so-called delta sign (**Figure 1**). When contrast is administered, the obstructed sinus reveals itself as an empty triangle, which may not be visible in the first few days after the onset but persists for several more weeks. Recent work confirms the high diagnostic efficacy of both CT venography and magnetic resonance venography (MRV) in the diagnosis of CVT [21, 23]. The visualization of small sinuses and small cerebral veins with low flow appears to be easier with CT venography than with MRV. The undoubted advantages of CT venography are the rapid image acquisition and the ability to perform the examination in patients with pacemakers or other ferromagnetic devices. The downside of CT is the exposure to ionizing radiation and the need to administer a shadowing agent. The advantages of MR are the ability to image a thrombus and the high sensitivity.

Currently, MR examination and MR venography with venous phase are the methods of choice for the diagnosis of CVT [5, 10, 18, 20, 21]. The resonance image of an obstructed vessel changes in different sequences depending on the 'age' of the

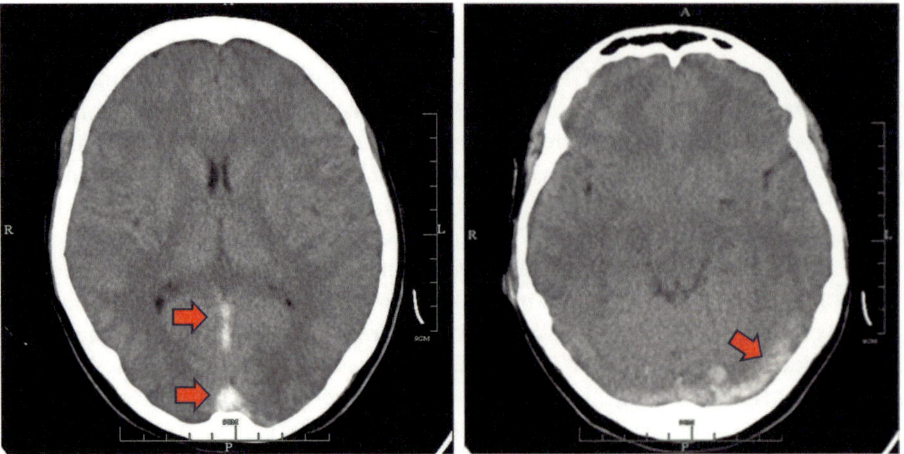

Figure 1.
Thrombosis in the superior sagittal sinus (delta sign), left straight and transverse sinus in non-contrast CT images: (Source: from the records of the Neurology Department with Stroke Unit of the Stanislaw Staszic Specialist Hospital in Piła).

thrombus. In the acute period, a newly formed thrombus reveals itself as an isointense signal in the T1 sequence and a hypointense signal in the T2 sequence, making differentiation from normal vessels difficult. Only after about 5 days from the onset of the illness does the obstructed sinus give a hyperintense signal on T1- and T2-weighted images [5, 22, 24]. The use of T2* and susceptibility weighted imaging (SWI) techniques increases the likelihood of visualizing obstructed veins, which is particularly useful in the first days of illness, in isolated cortical vein thrombosis, and when differentiating obstruction from hypoplasia [25]. In both SWI and T2*, thrombosis gives a hypointense signal. In MR venography (MRV), the Time of Flight (TOF) technique is the most commonly used, but shadowing can also be used [26]. **Figure 2** illustrates thrombosis in the superior sagittal sinus and cerebral veins on MR examination.

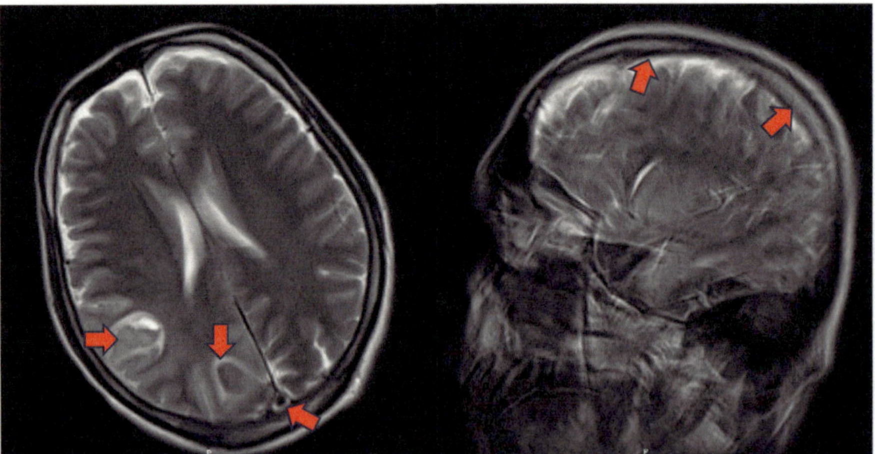

Figure 2.
MR image of venous thrombosis of the superior sagittal sinus and cerebral venous vessels: (Source: from the records of the Neurology Department with Stroke Unit of the Stanislaw Staszic Specialist Hospital in Piła).

Digital subtraction angiography (DSA) is the method with the highest sensitivity and specificity for the diagnosis of CVT but is only performed in doubtful cases due to the invasive nature of the examination [5, 10, 27]. DSA and MR angiography show a high level of concordance in their results [5].

Below are examples of neuroimaging studies in cerebral venous thrombosis:

3. Treatment

3.1 Acute treatment

3.1.1 Anticoagulant treatment

A meta-analysis of two studies using unfractionated heparin (UFH) or low-molecular-weight heparin (LMWH) in the treatment of CVT showed that the use of UFH or LMWH may have a beneficial effect on prognosis [28, 29]. However, due to the small number of cases (N = 79), statistical significance was not obtained for either the reduction in the risk of death or disability (RR 0.46; 95% CI: 0.16–1.31) or the reduction in the isolated risk of death (RR 0.33; 95% CI: 0.08–1.21). Importantly, no new symptomatic intracranial bleeding was detected in patients treated with heparins [30, 31]. Notwithstanding the small number of patients involved and statistical limitations, these studies formed the basis for establishing EFNS and AAN recommendations in favor of the use of heparins in CVT [5, 10, 15, 18, 32].

Therapy with heparin at therapeutic doses is therefore recommended in the acute period of CVT. The recommendation also applies to cases with the presence of intracranial hemorrhage in the course of the disease [5, 10, 15, 18, 32].

3.2 Choice of heparin in acute CVT

One randomized trial comparing the efficacy and safety of UFH vs. LMWH is available [31]. The study involved 66 adults with CVT. Of the 32 patients randomized to UFH, six (19%) died, while there were no deaths in the group of 34 patients receiving LMWH (RR LMWH vs. UFH, 0.073; 95% CI, 0.0043–1.24). The group treated with LMWH was more likely to experience a complete recovery after 3 months (RR, 1.37; 95% CI, 1.02–1.83). Serious hemorrhagic (extracerebral) complications were observed in 3 patients treated with UFH and did not occur in patients in the LMWH group (RR, 0.13; 95% CI, 0.0072–2.51). Similar results were obtained by Continho et al. [33].

It is suggested that anticoagulant treatment in the acute period should be provided with LMWH rather than UFH. This recommendation does not apply to patients with contraindications to LMWH (e.g., renal failure) or situations where rapid reversal of the anticoagulant effect may be necessary (e.g., planned neurosurgical intervention). LMWH is recommended at a therapeutic dose of 2 x daily 0.1 IU per kg body weight for 1–3 weeks [5, 10, 15, 18, 32].

3.3 Endovascular thrombolysis and thrombectomy

Mechanical thrombectomy and/or targeted thrombolysis are potential therapeutic options for patients in whom anticoagulation treatment has failed. Thrombolytic treatment involves the administration of a drug [urokinase, streptokinase, or recombinant tissue plasminogen activator (rtPA)] locally after the thrombus has been accessed with a microcatheter. Mechanical thrombectomy can be performed using dedicated systems, balloon angioplasty, non-expandable stents, or a combination of these methods [34]. Unfortunately, there are no randomized study results available in this area. Many case reports and systematic reviews have been published, suggesting a potential benefit of thrombolytic and/or endovascular treatment in selected patients [34–38]. In the majority of cases described, the thrombolytic drug was urokinase (73%), less frequently streptokinase, and rtPA. Complete or partial recanalization was achieved in 62% of cases, and 88% of patients maintained full independence (in Modified Ranking *Scale* (mRS) - 0–2 points). Intracranial bleeding occurred in 12% of the treated patients (2 out of 3 fatal) and extracranial bleeding in 19% of them (none of them fatal).

In a systematic review on thrombectomy (N = 185) with eventual subsequent thrombolysis (75% of cases), complete or partial recanalization was achieved in 95% of treated patients, and full independence (mRS 0–2) was achieved in 84% of them. Intracranial hemorrhage was the main complication (10%) [37]. Despite the high average rate of recanalization and favorable prognosis, the epidemiological and methodological heterogeneity of individual studies, as well as the potential for systematic bias, should be considered. The Thrombolysis or Anticoagulation for Cerebral Venous Thrombosis study (TO-ACT study) evaluating the efficacy and safety of endovascular treatment (EVT) performed after 1 year showed that the use of thrombectomy in CVT combined with standard medical care did not improve patients' functional status [39]. Perhaps future studies will show better recovery rates after EVT in this patient population [39].

This therapeutic option can be used in a precisely selected group of patients, high-risk patients with significant deterioration despite standard treatment, after exclusion of other causes of deterioration. This treatment can be carried out in specialized centers that provide interventional stroke treatment [5, 15, 40].

4. Length of anticoagulant treatment

The risk of recurrence of both subsequent CVT and other thromboembolic events is relatively low and amounts to 2–3% for recurrent CVT and 3–8% for extracerebral events. Most recurrent incidents occur within the first year of onset [5, 11, 41].

When the cause of thrombosis is a transient factor (e.g., pregnancy, puerperium, infection), anticoagulant treatment with an oral anticoagulant is continued for 3–6 months, whereas in idiopathic thrombosis it is continued for 6–12 months [5, 10, 15, 18].

Patients with recurrent incidents of venous thrombosis and those with a thrombophilic hypercoagulable state with a high risk of thrombosis require continuous anticoagulation [5, 10, 15, 18].

5. Novel oral anticoagulants (NOACs, direct oral anticoagulants (DOACs)) in the treatment of CVT

In the acute phase of CVT, antithrombotic treatment aims to prevent thrombus development, facilitate recanalization, and then, prevent recurrence.

After the acute phase of treatment for cerebral venous thrombosis, long-term treatment with an oral anticoagulant is initiated. Vitamin K antagonists (VKAs) are available and still widely used as continuation therapy after the acute phase of CVT, while direct oral anticoagulants (DOACs), which are direct inhibitors of individual coagulation factors, are also an option. The latter can also be used for oral anticoagulant therapy in patients without contraindications [5, 18].

Several single-case studies are available, as well as randomized trials of the use of DOACs in CVT [42–48]. In an international prospective study with the acronym RE-SPECT CVT, 120 CVT patients were randomized in a 1:1 ratio, where one group received warfarin under international normalized ratio (INR) control (INR was maintained at 2–3), while the other group received dabigatran at a dose of 2x150 mg. Oral anticoagulants were introduced 5–15 days after the initial heparin anticoagulant therapy, and treatment was continued for 6 months. No recurrent incidents of venous thromboembolism occurred in any of the groups. Regarding major bleeding after treatment with an oral anticoagulant, there was one gastrointestinal bleed in the dabigatran-treated group (1.7% [95% CI, 0.0–8.9%]) and two intracerebral hemorrhages in the warfarin-treated group (3.3% [95% CI, 0.4–11.5%]) [46]. In contrast, in the Study of Rivaroxaban in Cerebral Venous Thrombosis (SECRET study), 53 patients with cerebral venous thrombosis were randomized in a 1:1 ratio, with one group receiving rivaroxaban at a dose of 20 mg per day, compared to warfarin at a dose ensuring an INR value of 2–3. Nineteen of 26 patients in the rivaroxaban group received the drug ≤4 days of initial parenteral anticoagulant therapy. After 6 months, there was only one incident of recurrent cerebral venous thrombosis and one intracerebral hemorrhage (3.8% [95% CI, 01–19.6%]) in the rivaroxaban group with no recurrent thrombotic incidents or bleeding in the control group [47]. A large retrospective international study, Direct oral anticoagulants versus warfarin in the treatment of cerebral venous thrombosis with the acronym ACTIO-CVT compared the incidence of adverse events in 845 CVT patients who were prescribed a VKA or DOAC as part of routine clinical care between 2015 and 2020. The DOACs used included apixaban (67%), rivaroxaban (18%), and dabigatran (14%), or different DOACs (3%). This study showed no significant difference in the rate of recurrent venous thromboembolism (adjusted risk ratio 0.94 [95% CI, 0.15–1.73]). The risk of major hemorrhage was lower in the DOAC group (adjusted risk ratio, 0.35 [95% CI, 0.15–0.82]) [48]. No differences in recanalization rates between groups were observed [48].

All the presented studies excluded individuals with malignant tumors, antiphospholipid syndrome, and pregnant women. [46–48].

It should be noted that dabigatran, like rivaroxaban and apixaban, cannot be used in pregnant women [5, 18, 46–48]. In addition, drugs from this group are not recommended in antiphospholipid syndrome, where vitamin K antagonists (acenocoumarol, warfarin) should be used under the control of the international normalized ratio (INR) (INR should be kept at 2–3) [5, 18]. Administration of DOACs is carried out according to the established guidelines for this class of drugs and requires close monitoring of the patient [5, 18].

6. Treatment of increased intracranial pressure

Increased intracranial pressure is a common complication of acute CVT and is a major cause of death [14]. The predominant symptom is headache with or without swelling of the second cranial nerve = optic nerve (CNII) disc. Edema management should include appropriate positioning of the patient with the head elevated, controlled hyperventilation to reduce the partial pressure of carbon dioxide in arterial blood to 30–35 mmHg, and continuous monitoring of visual acuity. Edema of minor severity is reduced by anticoagulant treatment. Diuretics from the carbonic anhydrase inhibitor group, such as acetazolamide, which reduces intracranial pressure by decreasing cerebrospinal fluid production, are often used, thereby reducing headaches and preventing vision loss [49, 50]. The effect of this treatment is usually insufficient [49]. Seventeen studies have been identified in which acetazolamide was used with beneficial effects; these are case studies or review papers. To date, there is little research confirming the effect of carbonic anhydrase inhibitors and diuretics on headache and visual loss in CVT [18, 49]. It has been shown that acetazolamide in idiopathic central cranial hypertension with moderate headache and visual impairment in combination with a low-sodium diet has a beneficial effect on visual field improvement [49].

Experts believe that in cases of isolated intracranial hypertension in the course of CVT with severe headache and deterioration of visual acuity, acetazolamide therapy can be considered if its use is deemed safe [5, 18].

Steroids.

Steroids may be used in patients with acute CVT only with coexisting inflammatory connective tissue diseases (e.g., Behcet's disease, systemic lupus), as they improve the outcome of treatment. However, steroids should not be used in patients without these connective tissue disorders, as they then do not improve outcomes and do not prevent death [5, 10, 18, 50, 51].

7. Therapeutic puncture

In patients with symptoms of intracranial hypertension with severe headache, swelling of the CNII discs, and deterioration of visual acuity, intracranial hypertension can be reduced by therapeutic lumbar puncture [5, 10, 18, 52–54]. However, the effect of lumbar puncture is short-lived and requires discontinuation of anticoagulant treatment. Therefore, it is suggested that lumbar puncture be performed in emergency situations, with threatening loss of vision. Then the prevention of impending blindness outweighs the low risk of complications. Patients with compromised vision usually require a neurosurgical drainage procedure [18, 55].

Therapeutic lumbar puncture may be performed in patients with intracranial hypertension in the course of CVT if it can help to inhibit vision loss or significantly contribute to headache reduction, provided the safety profile is acceptable [5, 10, 18].

8. Valvular system/cerebrospinal fluid drainage

Hydrocephalus is an uncommon complication of CVT and is usually present in cases of deep vein thrombosis, posterior cranial cavity lesions, or intraventricular hemorrhage [55, 56]. It is suggested that cerebrospinal fluid drainage should not be routinely performed in patients with acute CVT and impending herniation due to the lack of convincing evidence for its efficacy [5, 10, 18].

8.1 Surgical decompression

Herniation due to mass effect is the leading cause of death in patients during the acute phase of CVT [57]. Hemicraniectomy is the procedure of choice in life-threatening cases of rapidly increasing edema and threatening herniation, with acutely increasing disturbance of consciousness, with (or without) symptoms of third nerve palsy. Based on the available case studies, two systematic reviews, and the results of non-randomized studies [57–60] comparing outcomes with and without decompression, it is apparent that surgical decompression can prevent deaths due to CVT and significantly reduce the proportion of patients with severe disability. The mortality rate in patients who underwent decompression was 19%, the rate of severe disability was 3%, and complete recovery was achieved in 31% of patients. Good treatment outcomes were observed even in advanced stages of herniation [59, 60]. A worse prognosis was observed in patients in a coma with bilateral central nervous system damage.

European Stroke Organization (ESO) experts strongly recommend hemicraniectomy as a life-saving procedure in patients with CVT and massive edema [5, 18].

8.2 Epileptic seizures

Epileptic seizures in CVT are observed in 37% of adult patients with CVT [10]. Factors that increase the risk of seizures are the presence of supranuclear lesions, cortical vein thrombosis, superior sagittal sinus thrombosis, and perianal thrombosis [61, 62]. Some studies indicate a relationship between the occurrence of seizures during the acute phase of the disease and mortality [63]. A reduction in the risk of early seizures with treatment has also been confirmed in patients with supranuclear lesions and early seizures (OR, 0.0006; CI, 0.001–0.05) [62].

Based on American Heart Academy (AHA) recommendations, antiepileptic drugs (AEDs) are recommended for patients with supratentorial lesions and early seizures; treatment is not recommended for patients without seizures [5, 10]. European guidelines recommend the use of AEDs in patients with early seizures and a hemorrhagic focus [18, 32, 63].

The use of antiepileptic drugs in patients in the acute period of CVT after an episode of seizures, with the presence of supratentorial lesions, prevents early recurrence of epileptic seizures [62]. It has been suggested that the dose of AEDs can be reduced after 3–6 months if no further seizures have occurred [18, 32, 52].

9. Cerebral venous thrombosis in pregnancy

Pregnancy and the postpartum period promote hypercoagulability. The incidence rate of cerebral venous thrombosis during pregnancy is very high at 11.6/100,000 pregnancies, accounting for more than half (57%) of all strokes among pregnant women (136/240). The highest risk of incidence is in the third trimester of pregnancy and the first 4 weeks of postpartum (about 70%). Cesarean section, prolonged hospitalization, and older maternal age further increase the risk of CVT [2, 22, 64]. Studies confirm the favorable outcome of treatment during pregnancy and postpartum with low-molecular-weight heparins administered subcutaneously [31, 65–69].

Treatment during pregnancy should be carried out with low-molecular-weight heparins and during the postpartum period, with low-molecular-weight heparins or vitamin K antagonists (INR should then be kept at 2–3). The total duration of treatment should not be less than 6 months [5, 10, 18]. In contrast, oral anticoagulants from the DOAC group should not be used in pregnancy and the postpartum period [5, 18, 46–48, 70].

9.1 Contraception after CVT

The results of published studies and a systematic review confirm that the use of oral contraceptives carries a high risk of CVT (OR = 7.59, 95% CI 3.82–15.09) [71]. This risk may be higher with the coexistence of other conditions causing hypercoagulability. There is also a lack of data on the effect of duration of contraceptive use or the use of progestogen-only contraception.

It is suggested that women of childbearing age should not take oral contraceptives after a CVT incident. Women must be informed of the increased risk of CVT associated with contraceptive use [5, 10, 18].

9.2 CVT and subsequent pregnancy

Previous CVT incidents and thrombosis during pregnancy and the postpartum period are not contraindications for subsequent pregnancies [5, 10, 18]. In a systematic review of the literature (13 studies, 217 pregnancies), a recurrence of CVT was observed in 0.5% of cases and an extramedullary thrombotic incident, in 3% of cases [69, 70].

Women with a history of CVT should be informed of the possible risk of thromboembolic events in a subsequent pregnancy; however, a history of venous cerebral thrombosis is not a contraindication to a subsequent pregnancy [5, 10, 18].

Results from a meta-analysis of randomized studies evaluating the safety and efficacy of anticoagulant prophylaxis in pregnant women with a history of thromboembolic events other than cerebral thrombosis suggest a benefit from its use (although not reaching statistical significance), and it was not associated with a significant increase in hemorrhagic complications [70]. In addition, the use of thromboprophylaxis has been shown to result in fewer miscarriages in pregnant women (11% of pregnant women with prophylaxis vs. 19% of pregnant women without prophylaxis) [69, 70]. ESO/EAN recommend prophylaxis with low-molecular-weight heparins during pregnancy and the postpartum period in women after a CVT incident, in the absence of contraindications to such treatment [5, 10, 15, 18].

10. Conclusions

Cerebral venous thrombosis may be suspected in patients with unexplained severe headaches accompanied by epileptic seizures and various focal symptoms, especially if conditions predisposing to thrombosis, such as pregnancy, childbirth, the postpartum period, use of oral contraceptives, thrombophilia, obesity, infections (especially COVID-19), certain types of thrombocytopenia, or if these symptoms occur in a young woman (a demographic factor), are present.

The recommended test to confirm the diagnosis is MR/MRV, but in centers with limited capacity to perform it, CT and angio-CT with venous phase can be an alternative.

In the acute phase of CVT, heparin is used, with a preference for low-molecular-weight heparin at a therapeutic dose. This is followed by transitioning to oral anticoagulants, which are administered for 3–12 months depending on the cause, or indefinitely in cases of severe thrombophilia or recurrent venous thromboembolism. As far as oral anticoagulants are concerned, in addition to vitamin K antagonists, DOACs can also be safely used according to the current guidelines (they cannot be used in pregnancy and postpartum periods or in antiphospholipid syndrome). Endovascular treatment is reserved only for specific patients (those with features of clot propagation, or when neurological status worsens despite conservative treatment, or when there are contraindications to anticoagulant therapy), preferably in centers with experience in this type of therapy. Decompressive neurosurgical procedures are considered a life-saving intervention in cases of significant brain edema that does not respond to conservative treatment.

Women with CVT during pregnancy are treated with full-dose LMWH throughout pregnancy, and, after delivery, they can be switched to an oral anticoagulant from the vitamin K antagonist group with a target INR of 2.0 to 3.0; this treatment should be continued for at least 6 weeks after delivery. Having experienced CVT is not a contraindication to a subsequent pregnancy. Prophylaxis with LMWH during pregnancy and in the postpartum period is then indicated.

It is also important to remember that, although rarely, a few days or weeks after the adenovirus-based SARS-CoV-2 vaccine, headache and thrombocytopenia with concurrent CVT may occur. In such cases, consultation with a hematologist is necessary, and treatment is carried out in collaboration with the hematologist.

Author details

Małgorzata Wiszniewska[1,2]

1 Medical Rescue Department, Stanisław Staszic State University of Applied Sciences, Piła, Poland

2 Neurological Department with Stroke Unit, Stanisław Staszic Specialist Hospital, Piła, Poland

*Address all correspondence to: mpwisz@gmail.com

References

[1] Bousser M-G, Ferro JM. Cerebral venous thrombosis: An update. Lancet Neurology. 2007;**6**(2):162-170. DOI: 10.1016/S1474-4422(07)70029-7

[2] Coutinho JM, Zuurbier SM, Aramideh M, et al. The incidence of cerebral venous thrombosis: A cross-sectional study. Stroke. 2012;**43**(12):3375-3377. DOI: 10.1161/STROKEAHA.112.671453

[3] Ferro JM, Canhão P, Aguiar de Sousa D. Cerebral venous thrombosis. La Presse Médicale. 2016;**45**(12):e429-e450. DOI: 10.1016/j.lpm.2016.10.007

[4] Ferro JM, Canhão P, Bousser MG, et al. Cerebral vein and dural sinus thrombosis in elderly patients. Stroke. 2005;**36**(9):1927-1932. DOI: 10.1161/01.STR.0000177894.05495.54

[5] Saposnik G, Bushnell C, Coutinho JM, et al. Diagnosis and management of cerebral venous thrombosis: A scientific statement from the American Heart Association. Stroke. 2024;**55**:e77-e90

[6] Lauw M, Barco S, Coutinho J, et al. Cerebral venous thrombosis and thrombophilia: A systematic review and meta-analysis. Seminars in Thrombosis and Hemostasis. 2013;**39**(8):913-927. DOI: 10.1055/s-0033-1357504

[7] Saadatnia M, Salehi M, Movahedian A, et al. Factor V Leiden, factor V Cambridge, factor II GA20210, and methylenetetrahydrofolate reductase in cerebral venous and sinus thrombosis: A case-control study. Journal of Research in Medical Sciences : The Official Journal of Isfahan University of Medical Sciences. 2015;**20**(6):554-562. DOI: 10.4103/1735-1995.165956

[8] Marjot T, Yadav S, Hasan N, et al. Genes associated with adult cerebral venous thrombosis. Stroke. 2011;**42**(4):913-918. DOI: 10.1161/STROKEAHA.110.602672

[9] Zuurbier SM, Arnold M, Middeldorp S, et al. Risk of cerebral venous thrombosis in obese women. JAMA Neurology. 2016;**73**:579-584. DOI: 10.1001/jamaneurol.2016.0001

[10] Saposnik G, Barinagarrementeria F, Brown RD Jr, et al. Diagnosis and management of cerebral venous thrombosis: A statement for healthcare professionals from the American Heart Association/American Stroke Association. Stroke. 2011;**42**:1158-1192. DOI: 10.1161/STR.0b013e31820a8364

[11] Palazzo P, Agius P, Ingrand P, et al. Venous thrombotic recurrence after cerebral venous thrombosis: A long-term follow-up study. Stroke. 2017;**48**(2):321-326. DOI: 10.1161/STROKEAHA.116.015294

[12] King A, Doyle KM. Implications of COVID-19 to stroke medicine: An epidemiological and pathophysiological perspective. Current Vascular Pharmacology. 2022;**20**:333-340. DOI: 10.2174/1570161120666220428101337

[13] Dentali F, Poli D, Scoditti U, et al. Long-term outcomes of patients with cerebral vein thrombosis: A multicenter study. Journal of Thrombosis and Haemostasis. 2012;**10**(7):1297-1302. DOI: 10.1111/j.1538-7836.2012.04774

[14] Ferro JM, Canhao P, Stam J, et al. Prognosis of cerebral vein and dural sinus thrombosis: Results of the international study on cerebral vein and dural sinus thrombosis (ISCVT). Stroke.

2004;**35**:664-670. DOI: 10.1161/01.STR.0000117571.76197.26

[15] Aamodt AH, Skattor TH. Cerebral venous thrombosis. Seminars in Thrombosis and Hemostasis. 2022;**48**(3):309-317. DOI: 10.1055/s-0042-1742738

[16] Coutinho JM. Cerebral venous thrombosis. Journal of Thrombosis and Haemostasis. 2015;**13**(S1):S238-S244. DOI: 10.1111/jth.12945

[17] Ferro JM, Canhão P, Stam J, et al. Delay in the diagnosis of cerebral vein and dural sinus thrombosis: Influence on outcome. Stroke; A Journal of Cerebral Circulation. 2009;**40**(9):3133-3138. DOI: 10.1161/STROKEAHA.109.553891

[18] Ferro JM, Bousser M-G, Canhão P, et al. European stroke organization guideline for the diagnosis and treatment of cerebral venous thrombosis - Endorsed by the European Academy of Neurology. European Journal of Neurology. 2017;**24**(10):1203-1213. DOI: 10.1111/ene.13381

[19] Appenzeller S, Zeller CB, Annichino-Bizzachi JM, et al. Cerebral venous thrombosis: Influence of risk factors and imaging findings on prognosis. Clinical Neurology and Neurosurgery. 2005;**107**(5):371-378. DOI: 10.1016/j.clineuro.2004.10.004

[20] Gao L, Xu W, Li T, et al. Accuracy of magnetic resonance venography in diagnosing cerebral venous sinus thrombosis. Thrombosis Research. 2018;**167**:64-73. DOI: 10.1016/j.thromres.2018.05.012

[21] Xu W. The performance of CT versus MRI in the differential diagnosis of cerebral venous thrombosis. Thrombosis and Haemostasis. 2018;**118**(6):1067-1077. DOI: 10.1055/s-0038-1642636

[22] Bonneville F. Imaging of cerebral venous thrombosis. Diagnostic and Interventional Imaging. 2014;**95**(12):1145-1150. DOI: 10.1016/j.diii.2014.10.006

[23] Ferro JM, Canhão P. Cerebral venous sinus thrombosis: Update on diagnosis and management. Current Cardiology Reports. 2014;**16**(9). Article: 523. DOI: 10.1007/s11886-014-0523-2

[24] Leach JL, Strub WM, Gaskill-Shipley MF. Cerebral venous thrombus signal intensity and susceptibility effects on gradient recalled-echo MR imaging. American Journal of Neuroradiology. 2007;**28**(5):940-945

[25] Boukobza M, Crassard I, Bousser MG, et al. MR imaging features of isolated cortical vein thrombosis: Diagnosis and follow-up. American Journal of Neuroradiology. 2009;**30**(2):344-348. DOI: 10.3174/ajnr.A1332

[26] Agid R, Shelef I, Scott JN, et al. Imaging of the intracranial venous system. The Neurologist. 2008;**14**(1):12-22. DOI: 10.1097/NRL.0b013e318157f791

[27] Wong GKC, Siu DYW, Abrigo JM, et al. Computed tomographic angiography and venography for young or nonhypertensive patients with acute spontaneous intracerebral hemorrhage. Stroke. 2011;**42**(1):211-213. DOI: 10.1161/STROKEAHA.110.592337

[28] De Bruijn SFTM, Stam J. Randomized, placebo controlled trial of anticoagulant treatment with low molecular weighted heparin for cerebral venous thrombosis. Stroke. 1999;**30**(3):484-488. DOI: 10.1161/01.str.30.3.484

[29] Einhupl KM, Villringer A, Mehraein S, et al. Heparin treatment

in sinus venous thrombosis. The Lancet. 1991;**338**(8767):597-600. DOI: 10.1016/0140-6736(91)90607-Q

[30] Coutinho J, de Bruijn SF, Deveber G, et al. Anticoagulation for cerebral venous sinus thrombosis. Cochrane Database of Systematic Reviews. 2011;(8):CD002005 (Online). DOI: 10.1002/14651858.CD002005.pub2

[31] Misra UK, Kalita J, Chandra S, et al. Low molecular weight heparin versus unfractionated heparin in cerebral venous sinus thrombosis: A randomized controlled trial. European Journal of Neurology. 2012;**19**(7):1030-1036. DOI: 10.1111/j.1468-1331.2012.03690

[32] Ferro JM, de Sousa DA. Cerebral venous thrombosis: An update. Cerebral venous thrombosis. Current Neurology and Neuroscience Reports. 2019;**19**(10):74. DOI: 10.1007/s11910-019-0988

[33] Coutinho JM, Ferro JM, Canhão P, et al. Unfractionated or low-molecular weight heparin for the treatment of cerebral venous thrombosis. Stroke. 2010;**41**(11):2575-2580. DOI: 10.1161/STROKEAHA.110.588822

[34] Goyal M, Fladt J, Coutinho JM, et al. Endovascular treatment for cerebral venous thrombosis: Current status, challenges, and opportunities. Journal of Neurointerventional Surgery. 2022;**14**(8):788-793

[35] Haghighi AB, Mahmoodi M, Edgell RC, et al. Mechanical thrombectomy for cerebral venous sinus thrombosis: A comprehensive literature review. Clinical and Applied Thrombosis/Hemostasis. 2014;**20**(5):507-515. DOI: 10.1177/1076029612470968

[36] Nyberg EM, Case D, Nagae LM, et al. The addition of endovascular intervention for dural venous sinus thrombosis: Single-center experience and review of literature. Journal of Stroke and Cerebrovascular Diseases : The Official Journal of National Stroke Association. 2017;**80**:51. DOI: 10.1016/j.jstrokecerebrovasdis.2017.05.006

[37] Siddiqui FM, Dandapat S, Banerjee C, et al. Mechanical thrombectomy in cerebral venous thrombosis. Stroke. 2015;**46**(5):1263-1268. DOI: 10.1161/STROKEAHA.114.007465

[38] Viegas LD, Stolz E, Canhão P, et al. Systemic thrombolysis for cerebral venous and dural sinus thrombosis: A systematic review. Cerebrovascular Diseases. 2014;**37**(1):43-50. DOI: 10.1159/000356840

[39] Coutinho JM, Zuurbier SM, Bousse M-G, Ji X, et al. Effect of endovascular treatment with medical management vs standard care on severe cerebral venous thrombosis: The TO-ACT randomized clinical trial. JAMA Neurology. 2020;**77**(8):966-973

[40] Ageno W, Beyer-Westendorf J, Garcia DA, et al. Guidance for the management of venous thrombosis in unusual sites. Journal of Thrombosis and Thrombolysis. 2016;**41**(1):129-143. DOI: 10.1007/s11239-015-1308-1

[41] Miranda B, Aaron S, Arauz A, et al. The benefit of extending oral anticoagulation treatment (EXCOA) after acute cerebral vein thrombosis (CVT): EXCOA-CVT cluster randomized trial protocol. International Journal of Stroke. 2018;**13**(7):771-774. DOI: 10.1177/1747493018778137

[42] Geisbüsch C, Richter D, Herweh C, et al. Novel factor Xa inhibitor for the treatment of cerebral venous and sinus thrombosis: First experience in 7

patients. Stroke. 2014;**45**(8):2469-2471. DOI: 10.1161/STROKEAHA.114.006167

[43] Mendonça MD, Barbosa R, Cruz-e-Silva V, et al. Oral direct thrombin inhibitor as an alternative in the management of cerebral venous thrombosis: A series of 15 patients. International Journal of Stroke. 2015;**10**(7):1115-1118. DOI: 10.1111/ijs.12462

[44] Nepal G, Kharel S, Bhagat R, et al. Safety and efficacy of direct oral anticoagulants in cerebral venous thrombosis: A meta-analysis. Acta Neurologica Scandinavica. 2022;**145**(1):10-23

[45] Cohen O, Pegoraro S, Ageno W. Cerebral venous thrombosis. Minerva Medica. 2021;**112**(6):755-766. DOI: 10.23736/S0026-4806.21.07353-5

[46] Ferro JM, Coutinho JM, Dentali F, et al. Safety and efficacy of dabigatran etexilate vs dose-adjusted warfarin in patients with cerebral venous thrombosis: A randomized clinical trial. JAMA Neurology. 2019;**76**:1457-1465. DOI: 10.1001/jamaneurol.2019.2764

[47] Field T, Dizonno V, Almekhlafi MA, Bala F, et al. Study of rivaroxaban in cerebral venous thrombosis: A randomized controlled feasibility trial comparing anticoagulation with rivaroxaban to standard-of- care in symptomatic cerebral venous thrombosis. Stroke. 2023;**54**:2724-2736. DOI: 10.1161/STROKEAHA.123.044113

[48] Yaghi S, Shu L, Bakradze E, et al. Direct oral anticoagulants versus warfarin in the treatment of cerebral venous thrombosis (ACTION-CVT): A multicenter international study. Stroke. 2022;**53**:728-738. DOI: 10.1161/STROKEAHA.121.037541

[49] Wall M, McDermott MP, Kieburtz KD, et al. NORDIC idiopathic intracranial hypertension study group writing committee. Effect of acetazolamide on visual function in patients with idiopathic intracranial hypertension and mild visual loss: The idiopathic intracranial hypertension treatment trial. JAMA. 2014;**311**:1641-1651

[50] Canhão P, Cortesão A, Cabral M, et al. Are steroids useful to treat cerebral venous thrombosis? Stroke. 2008;**39**(1):105-110. DOI: 10.1161/STROKEAHA.107.484089

[51] De Sousa DA, Mestre T, Ferro JM. Cerebral venous thrombosis in Behçet's disease: A systematic review. Journal of Neurology. 2011;**258**(5):719-727. DOI: 10.1007/s00415-010-5885-9

[52] Coutinho JM, Middeldorp S. Advances in the treatment of cerebral venous thrombosis. 2014;**16**:299. DOI: 10.1007/s11940-014-0299-0

[53] Canhão P, Abreu LF, Ferro JM, et al. ISCVT investigators. Safety of lumbar puncture in patients with cerebral venous thrombosis. European Journal of Neurology. 2013;**20**:1075-1080

[54] Zuurbier S, Couthinho J. Cerebral venous thrombosis. Advances in Experimental Medicine and Biology. 2017;**906**:183-193. DOI: 10.1007/5584

[55] Zuurbier SM, van den Berg R, Troost D, et al. Hydrocephalus in cerebral venous thrombosis. Journal of Neurology. 2015;**262**(4):931-937. DOI: 10.1007/s00415-015-7652-4

[56] Canhão P, Ferro JM, Lindgren AG, et al. Causes and predictors of death in cerebral venous thrombosis. Stroke. 2005;**36**(8):1720-1725. DOI: 10.1161/01.STR.0000173152.84438.1c

[57] Théaudin M, Crassard I, Bresson D, et al. Should decompressive surgery be performed in malignant cerebral venous thrombosis?: A series of 12 patients. Stroke. 2010;**41**(4):727-731. DOI: 10.1161/STROKEAHA.109.572909

[58] Ferro JM, Crassard I, Coutinho JM, et al. Decompressive surgery in cerebrovenous thrombosis: A multicenter registry and a systematic review of individual patient data. Stroke. 2011;**42**(10):2825-2831. DOI: 10.1161/STROKEAHA.111.615393

[59] Raza E, Shamim MS, Wadiwala MF, et al. Decompressive surgery for malignant cerebral venous sinus thrombosis: A retrospective case series from Pakistan and comparative literature review. Journal of Stroke and Cerebrovascular Diseases. 2014;**23**(1):e13-e22

[60] Zuurbier SM, Coutinho JM, Majoie CBLM, et al. Decompressive hemicraniectomy in severe cerebral venous thrombosis: A prospective case series. Journal of Neurology. 2012;**259**(6):1099-1105. DOI: 10.1007/s00415-011-6307-3

[61] Fam D, Saposnik G. Critical care management of cerebral venous thrombosis. Current Opinion in Critical Care. 2016:**22**(2):113-119. DOI: 10.1097/MCC.0000000000000278

[62] Ferro JM, Canhão P, Bousser MG, et al. Early seizures in cerebral vein and dural sinus thrombosis: Risk factors and role of antiepileptics. Stroke. 2008;**39**(4):1152-1158. DOI: 10.1161/STROKEAHA.107.487363

[63] Price M, Günther A, Tiwari D, et al. Antiepileptic drugs for the primary and secondary prevention of seizures after intracranial venous thrombosis. Cochrane Database of Systematic Reviews. 2014;**8**:1-14. DOI: 10.1002/14651858.CD008710.pub2

[64] Lanska DJ, Kryscio RJ. Risk factors for Peripartum and postpartum stroke and intracranial venous thrombosis. Stroke. 2000;**31**(6):1274-1282. DOI: 10.1161/01.STR.31.6.1274

[65] Demir CF, İnci MF, Özkan F, et al. Clinical and radiological management and outcome of pregnancies complicated by cerebral venous thrombosis: A review of 19 cases. Journal of Stroke and Cerebrovascular Diseases. 2013;**22**(8):1252-1257. DOI: 10.1016/j.jstrokecerebrovasdis.2012.07.004

[66] Coutinho JM, Ferro JM, Canhao P, et al. Cerebral venous and sinus thrombosis in women. Stroke. 2009;**40**:2356-2361. DOI: 10.1161/STROKEAHA.108.543884

[67] Fang T, Shu L, Elnazeir M, et al. Characteristics and outcomes of postpartum cerebral venous sinus thrombosis: A subgroup analysis of the ACTION-CVT study. Journal of Stroke and Cerebrovascular Diseases. 2022;**31**:106865. DOI: 10.1016/j.jstrokecerebrovasdis.2022.106865

[68] Kamel H, Navi BB, Sriram N, et al. Risk of a thrombotic event after the 6-week postpartum period. The New England Journal of Medicine. 2014;**370**:1307-1315. DOI: 10.1056/NEJMoa1311485

[69] Aguiar de Sousa D, Canhão P, Ferro JM. Safety of pregnancy after cerebral venous thrombosis: Systematic review update. Journal of Neurology. 2018;**265**:211-212. DOI: 10.1007/s00415-017-8666-x

[70] Bain E, Wilson A, Tooher R, et al. Prophylaxis for venous thromboembolic disease in pregnancy and the early

postnatal period. Cochrane Database of Systematic Reviews. 2014;**5**:CD001689. DOI: 10.1002/14651858.CD001689.pub2

[71] Amoozegar F, Ronksley PE, Sauve R, et al. Hormonal contraceptives and cerebral venous thrombosis risk: A systematic review and meta-analysis. Frontiers in Neurology. 2015;**6**:7. DOI: 10.3389/fneur.2015.00007